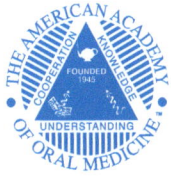

CLINICIAN'S GUIDE

Tobacco Cessation
THIRD EDITION

EDITORS

Abdel Rahim Mohammad, DDS, MS, MPH
Professor, Oral Medicine and Geriatric Dentistry Director of Tobacco Cessation and Community Outreach Programs College of Dentistry, formerly at The Ohio State University, College of Dentistry Columbus, Ohio

CONTRIBUTING AUTHORS

Ali Aboalela, BDS, MMEd, DMSc, FDS RCSEd
Consultant in Hospital Dentistry, Ministry of National Guard Health Affairs, Joint Appointtee Assistant Professor King Saud bin Abdulaziz University for Health Sciences

Ahmed Sultan, BDS, DABOM, FDS RCSEd
PHD candidate University of Maryland

Paul J. Vankevich, DMD, DABOM, FAGD, FICD
Formerly Tufts University, College of Dentistry

Contributing authors are members of the American Academy of Oral Medicine. This monograph represents a consensus of the contributing authors and not necessarily the private views of any of the individuals

CONTENTS

American Academy of Oral Medicine
2150 N. 107th St., Suite 205
Seattle, Washington 98133
TEL: (206) 209-5279
EMAIL: info@aaom.com   WEBSITE: www.aaom.com
©2017 American Academy of Oral Medicine

Notice

The authors and publisher have made every effort to ensure that the patient care recommended herein, including choice of drugs and drug dosages, is in accord with the accepted standard and practice at the time of publication. However, since research and regulation constantly change clinical standards, the reader is urged to check the product information sheet included in the package of each drug, which includes recommended doses, warnings, and contraindications. This is particularly important with new or infrequently used drugs. Any treatment regimen, particularly one involving medication, involves inherent risk that must be weighed on a case-by-case basis against the benefits anticipated. The reader is cautioned that the purpose of this book is to inform and enlighten; the information contained herein is not intended as, and should not be employed as, a substitute for individual diagnosis and treatment.

ISBN
Paperback: 978-1-936176-49-6
PDF: 978-1-936176-50-2

Printed in the United States

Notice: The authors and publisher have made every effort to ensure that the patient care recommended herein, including choice of drugs and drug dosages, is in accord with the accepted standard and practice at the time of publication. However, since research and regulation constantly change clinical standards, the reader is urged to check the product information sheet included in the package of each drug, which includes recommended doses, warnings, and contraindications. This is particularly important with new or infrequently used drugs. Any treatment regimen, particularly one involving medication, involves inherent risk that must be weighed on a case-by-case basis against the benefits anticipated. The reader is cautioned that the purpose of this book is to inform and enlighten; the information contained herein is not intended as, and should not be employed as, a substitute for individual diagnosis and treatment.

The Third edition of this Guide is dedicated to the memory of Jonathan A. Ship, DMD. Dr. Ship was an inspiration to a generation of students, oral medicine residents and colleagues and a revered member of the American Academy of Oral Medicine. His research contributions in geriatric dentistry, xerostomia, Sjögren's syndrome and oral, head and neck cancer will serve the professional community and society for generations. His friendship, guidance, professionalism and laughter are sorely missed by everyone who knew and loved him. Dr. Ship has contributed extensively to this Guide.

ABOUT THE AMERICAN ACADEMY OF ORAL MEDICINE (AAOM): The AAOM is a 501c6; nonprofit organization founded in 1945 as the American Academy of Dental Medicine and took its current name in 1966. The members of the American Academy of Oral Medicine include an internationally recognized group of health care professionals and experts concerned with the oral health care of patients who have complex medical conditions, oral mucosal disorders, and / or chronic orofacial pain. Oral Medicine is the field of dentistry concerned with the oral health care of medically complex patients and with the diagnosis and non-surgical management of medically-related disorders or conditions affecting the oral and maxillofacial region.

AMERICAN ACADEMY OF ORAL MEDICINE

MISSION:

1. To promote the study and dissemination of knowledge of the medical aspects of dentistry while serving the best interests of the public.

2. To promote the highest standards of care in the diagnosis and treatment of oral conditions that are not responsive to conventional dental or oral maxillofacial surgical procedures.

3. To provide an avenue of referral for dental practitioners who have patients with severe, life- threatening medical disorders or complex diagnostic problems involving the oral and maxillofacial region that require ongoing nonsurgical management.

4. To improve the quality of life of patients with medically related oral disease.

5. To foster increased understanding and cooperation between medical and dental professions.

6. To obtain American Dental Association recognition of oral medicine as a specialty.

The Academy achieves these goals by holding national meetings annually; by presenting lectures, workshops, and seminars; by sponsorship of the American Board of Oral Medicine; by the editorship of the Oral Medicine Section of *Oral Surgery, Oral Medicine, Oral Pathology, Oral Radiology*, and *Endodontics*; and by publishing monographs and position papers on timely subjects relating to oral medicine.

The presented information is based on current knowledge and accepted standards of practice. Following the guidelines set forth in this monograph may not ensure successful management of every patient. This monograph represents a consensus of the editors and authors and not necessarily the private views of any individual.

All brand name medications may have patents, service marks, trademarks, or registered trademarks and are the property of their respective companies.

This Clinician's Guide is another AAOM educational service.
Other Clinician's Guides available from the Academy include:

Treatment of Common Oral Conditions,
7/e Tobacco Cessation
Oral Health in Geriatric Patients, 3/e
Pharmacology, 2/e
Medically Complex Dental Patients 4/e
Salivary Gland & Chemosensory Disorders 1/e
Chronic Orofacial Pain 4/e

Preface

It is the position of the American Academy of Oral Medicine that there is no safe form of tobacco. The use of any tobacco product has an associated increased risk of oral and dental disease, systemic health problems, and the development of oral and oropharygeal cancer. The use of smokeless (spit) tobacco places the user at increased risk of oral cancer and a number of other noncancer oral conditions. Cigar use has been linked with cancer of the respiratory and upper aerodigestive tract and alveolar bone loss. All forms of tobacco adversely affect the periodontium and may result in premature tooth loss. All health care providers are urged to:

- ask every patient at every visit regarding their tobacco use,
- advise every tobacco using patient to quit,
- assess their readiness to quit,
- advise and assist in cessation when appropriate, and
- arrange for follow-up as necessary.

DENTAL PROVIDER TOBACCO INTERVENTION

The mission of the dental profession is to clinically apply knowledge and skill with the goal of optimizing a patient's oral health. The goals of the dental health care team are as follows:

- the prevention and treatment of orofacial and dental diseases and disorders with the objective of achieving optimum craniofacial health of the patient
- the result of professional dental care is an oral health status that enhances the overall
- wellness and quality of life of the patient
- to assist patients to achieve and maintain optimum oral health throughout their lives
- prevent premature tooth loss resulting in compromised nutritional health status
- prevent loss of function and degradation of appearance
- improve the patient's quality of life

Many preventable oral conditions and dental diseases have a significant effect on an individual's overall systemic health. By appropriately applying the principles of preventive dentistry, dental health care professionals can have a profound and positive impact on the health and well-being of patients. Preventive dentistry includes the interventions to prevent:

- dental caries
- periodontal disease
- oral and pharyngeal cancers
- occupational and athletic-related craniofacial injuries

The proper provision of clinical dental treatment is predicated upon an accurate diagnosis and an appropriate treatment plan. The goal of dentistry is to treat and prevent those diseases and disabilities that affect the teeth and oral structures by eliminating infection and restoring form and function. The susceptibility that a patient will incur a dental disease or condition is reflected in that patient's oral disease risk. Each patient should have the risk recognized and assessed, and that risk should be reduced or eliminated. Oral disease risk management is consistent with the goals of oral health promotion and preventive dentistry.

Dental health providers have a professional, ethical, and moral obligation to engage in tobacco prevention and treatment. Tobacco use in any form can adversely affect certain dental care and treatment prognoses, including wound healing, cosmetic dentistry and dental osseointegrated implants. Chronic tobacco use can cause oral and oropharyngeal cancer

Tobacco prevention, cessation, and treatment are the practical application of preventive dentistry. They are consistent with the goal of oral health promotion of helping patients attain and maintain optimum oral health. Tobacco use intervention should be a component of the dental treatment plan for all patients who use tobacco. The control of tobacco use by dental patients is consistent with the strategies of clinical risk assessment and management.

Standard Abbreviations

I	One	Prn	as needed (pro re nata)
ii	Two	Q	Every
iii	Three	q2h	every 2 hours
a	Before	q4h	every 4 hours
ac	before meals (ante cibum)	q6h	every 6 hours
ad lib	as desired (ad libitum)	q8h	every 8 hours
asap	as soon as possible	q12h	every 12 hours
AAOM	American Academy of Oral Medicine	Qam	every morning
bid	twice a day (bis in die)	Qd	every day (quaque die)
btl	Bottle	Qhs	every bedtime
c	With	Qid	four times a day (quarter in die)
cap	Capsule	Qod	every other day
CBC	complete blood count	Qpm	every evening
CDC	U. S. Center for Disease Control and Prevention	qsad	add a sufficient quantity to equal
crm	Cream	qwk	every week
disp	dispense on a prescription label	RAS	recurrent aphthous stomatitis
elix	Elixir	RAU	recurrent aphthous ulcer
FDA	U.S. Food and Drug Administration	RBC	red blood cell count
g	Gram	RHL	recurrent herpes labialis
gtt	Drop	RIH	recurrent intraoral herpes
h	Hour	Rx	Prescription
hs	at bedtime	s	Without
HSV	herpes simplex virus	Sig	patient dosing instructions on prescription label
IU	international units	Sol	Solution
IV	Intravenous	SPF	sun protection factor
L	Liter	stat	Immediately
liq	Liquid	Syr	Syrup
loz	Lozenge	Tab	Tablet
mg	Milligram	tbsp	Tablespoon
min	Minute	Tid	three times a day (ter in die)
mL	Milliliter	Top	Topical
NaF	sodium fluoride	Tsp	Teaspoon

Standard Abbreviations (*continued*)

Oint	Ointment	U	Unit
OTC	over-the-counter	ut dict	as directed (ut dictum)
Oz	Ounce	UV	Ultraviolet
P	After	Visc	Viscous
Pc	after meals	VZV	varicella-zoster virus
PABA	para-aminobenzoic acid	WBC	white blood cell count
PHN	postherpetic neuralgia	Wk	Week
PLT	platelet count	Yr	Year
Po	by mouth (per os)	Zn	Zinc

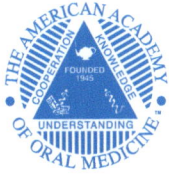

1 Tobacco Use and the Oral Health Professional

HISTORICAL BACKGROUND

Tobacco use has been part of our culture for centuries. It began with the discovery of the "New World" by Christopher Columbus. The explorers of the New World introduced the tobacco "habit" into Europe in the mid-1550s. Portuguese and Spanish sailors continued to spread this custom to the various ports in their trade routes and explorations. The Native Americans of North and South America believed that the tobacco plant had medicinal properties. This was the initial reason for introducing tobacco use into Europe. In Europe, tobacco was accepted as a true medical miracle and the tobacco products (ie, ointments, mouthrinses, pastes, poultices, and, of course, smoking) were used to treat a myriad of ailments. However, it was not very long before tobacco smoking was "recognized" as a health problem. In 1604, King James I warned his subjects that "the habit of smoking tobacco is disgusting to sight, repulsive to smell, dangerous to the brain, and noxious to the lung."

In 1859, a medical report on the hazardous effects of tobacco was published. A study of 68 patients in a hospital in Montpellier, France, who were diagnosed with cancers of the lips, tongue, tonsils, and other parts of the oral cavity revealed that all of the patients used tobacco. Sixty-six of the patients smoked the tobacco product in short-stemmed clay pipes. To decrease their risk from the continued use of tobacco, the patients switched to long-stemmed pipes rather than give up the habit.

Tobacco use in the form of cigarettes was nonexistent before the twentieth century. During the early twentieth century, tobacco use was primarily a male habit and chewing tobacco was the most popular form. Cigarette smoking did not begin to enter our society until 1913, when R. J. Reynolds introduced Camel brand , the first tobacco blended product. With cigarettes, the nicotine was inhaled into the lungs to achieve nicotine levels in the blood. The consumption of cigarettes increased quickly. This proved that aggressive advertising could create a demand and market for a product where there was no previous demand. By 1935, cigarette smoking was the prominent nicotine delivery system. This was the continued trend into the 1970s and 1980s. Today, tobacco is the single most preventable cause of disease and premature death in the world despite a decline in cigarette smoking from the year 2005-2014 (nearly 21 of every 100 adults to nearly 17 of every 100 adults).. Tobacco-related deaths will increase from 3 million per year in 1990 to 8.4 million per year in 2020. Thirty percent of all cancers can be attributed to tobacco use.

CONTEMPORARY TOBACCO USE

Modern tobacco use is prevalent and demographics of usage is constantly changing, The tobacco industry is constantly innovating, advertising and promoting new products that challenge the public health regulatory organizations to keep pace. The adverse effects of all forms of tobacco consumption affect all aspects of society. For example, tobacco use in the U.S. Military has been associated with training injuries, premature discharge, lower cardiovascular fitness and reduced troop readiness and increased costs for the Department of Defense (Smith, 2016).

Despite the known hazards of cigarette use, in 2016 according to the FDA Center for Tobacco products an estimated 42.1 million Americans—nearly one in five adults—currently smokecigarettes. Approximately one-third of all tobacco users in the United States will die prematurely because of their dependence on tobacco. On average, the inveterate one-pack per day smoker will lose 10 to 15 years of life expectancy.

In 2014 the US Department of Health and Human Services. *The Health Consequences of Smoking—50 Years of Progress. A Report of the Surgeon General.* reported that each year tobacco use kills more than 480,000 people in the United States.

Table 1 -1: Prevalence (%) of Cigarette Smoking in the Adult Population by US Region			
Region	Male	Female	Total N
Northeast			
Range	21.1–25.3	16.6–20.0	19.3–22
Media	23.2	18.3	20.6
Midwest			
Range	24.9–28.2	22.1–25.4	23.8–26.4
Median	26.5	23.7	25.1
South			
Range	24.6–27.9	18.4–21.3	21.7–24.0
Median	26.2	19.8	22.9
West			
Range	20.1–24.4	13.7–17.1	17.3–20.2
Median	22.2	15.4	18.7

The Substance Abuse and Mental Health Services Administration, Center for Behavioral Health Statistics and Quality in 2015 reported that each more than 2,600 U.S. youth under age 18 smoke their first cigarette, and nearly 600 become daily smokers.

In 2014 an estimated 42.1 million Americans—nearly one in five adults were cigarette smokers according to the Centers for Disease Control and Prevention, (Current Cigarette Smoking Among Adults – United States, 2005-2013. (MMWR. 2014;63:1108-1112.))

Recent data suggest that the individual who uses tobacco today may be more heavily dependent than in the past and that these individuals may also have a more difficult time quitting. Tobacco dependence affects the most socioeconomically disadvantaged members of society. In 2014, it was reported that only 5.4% of persons with a graduate degree (masters, professional, or doctorate) used tobacco, whereas 21.7% of those with a high school diploma and 43% with a general educational development (GED) degree used tobacco. Americans living below the poverty level have a higher smoking rate (26.3%) than those living at or above the poverty level (15.2%). A recent report stated that college students are using tobacco at a higher rate than previously reported. Two reports from the Surgeon General (1994 and 2012) showed that almost all smoking starts before the age of 18. Despite the sustained prevalence of tobacco use (Table 1-1), the response of the health care professions and the health care delivery systems has been disappointing. In the past part of this problem was be the fact that healthcare providers did not receive the appropriate training necessary to control tobacco use. Tobacco dependence education is not fully integrated into all U.S. and Canadian dental schools. A study revealed that dental school faculty was most confident in teaching tobacco-related pathology, but often lacked the interest and the skills needed to integrate tobacco dependence education into the curriculum and in patient care. (Davis) The current treatments available to treat tobacco dependence offer primary care providers a unique opportunity to reduce the morbidity and mortality associated with chronic tobacco use.

DENTAL PROVIDER TOBACCO INTERVENTION
The mission of the dental profession is to clinically apply knowledge and skill with the goal of optimizing a patient's oral health. The goal of the dental health care team is the prevention and treatment of orofacial and dental diseases and disorders with the objective of achieving optimum craniofacial health of the patient. The result of professional dental care is an oral health status that enhances the overall wellness and quality of life of the patient. The goal of the dental profession is to assist patients to achieve and maintain optimum oral health throughout their lives. Preventable premature tooth loss results in the loss of function and degradation of appearance and can profoundly affect the patient's quality of life. Many preventable oral conditions and dental diseases have a significant effect on an individual's overall systemic health. By appropriately applying the principles of preventive dentistry, dental health care professionals can have a profound and positive impact on the health and well-being of patients.

Preventive dentistry includes interventions to prevent dental caries, periodontal disease, oral and pharyngeal cancers, and sports-related craniofacial injuries. The proper provision of clinical dental treatment is predicated on an accurate diagnosis and an appropriate treatment plan. The goal of dentistry is to treat and prevent those diseases and disabilities that affect the teeth and oral structures by eliminating infection and restoring form and function. The susceptibility and likelihood that a patient will incur a dental disease or condition may be reflected in that patient's oral disease risk. Each patient should have his or her risk recognized and assessed, and that risk, ideally, should be reduced or eliminated. Oral disease risk management is consistent with the goals of oral health promotion and preventive dentistry.

Dental health providers have a professional, ethical, and moral obligation to engage in tobacco control. Tobacco use in any form (pyrolytic and topical) can adversely affect certain dental care and treatment prognoses, including wound healing, cosmetic dentistry, and dental osseointe-grated implants. Chronic tobacco use can cause oral and orophargeal cancer.

Tobacco prevention, cessation, and control are the practical application of preventive dentistry. They are consistent with the goal of oral health promotion of helping patients acquire and maintain optimum oral health. Tobacco use intervention should be part of the dental treatment plan of all patients who use tobacco. The control of tobacco use by dental patients is consistent with the evidence-based strategies of clinical risk assessment and management.

RATIONALE FOR ORAL HEALTH PROFESSIONAL INTERVENTION

Tobacco use in any form can adversely affect the oral cavity. In the United States, approximately 50% of adults and 75% of youth visit the dentist annually. Tobacco prevention and control is the practical application of comprehensive clinical dentistry. It is consistent with the goal of health promotion by helping patients attain and maintain optimum oral health. Identifying tobacco use as a dental problem is appropriate, and the intervention should be a component of the patient's comprehensive treatment plan. During a " teachable moment" in the course of a clinical patient encounter oral health care professionals can have a significant impact on a patient's decision to begin, continue, or quit using tobacco products.The purpose of this guideline is to highlight two concepts for the oral health care provider:

1. Tobacco use poses a significant overall health threat to our patients.
2. Tobacco dependence treatment delivered in a timely and effective manner (5 A's) will significantly reduce

the patient's risk of suffering from a tobacco-related disease, as outlined in Chapter 4, "Intervening with Tobacco Users."

We must consider that tobacco dependence has many features of a chronic disease, and failure to recognize this may undermine a clinician's motivation to treat tobacco use. Epidemiologic data have shown that more than 68% of the 40 million smokers in America were interested in quitting. The overall quit ratio in 2012 among adults was 55.1% with the greatest gains for those aged 65 years and older. By identifying every tobacco user, advising them to quit, assessing readiness to make an attempt, assisting with the quit attempt (setting a quit date, providing motivational literature and pharmacotherapy), and arranging for follow-up, the oral health care team will achieve 12 to 15% 1-year abstinence rates that, compared with the self-quit rate of 2 to 4%, are substantial. A recent study that investigated overcoming barriers to tobacco dependence treatment reported that of 100 smokers who try to quit without the help of their doctor, only five are abstinent one year later. Therefore, healthcare providers must consider the inadequacies of the health care system, the challenges of current attitudes, and the diagnostic and treatment protocols that result in a 95% failure rate in eliminating America's most deadly and modifiable risk factor.

TOBACCO USE IN THE UNITED STATES

Tobacco use continues to be a significant cause of death and disability in the United States. According to the Centers for Disease Control and Prevention, tobacco use is the leading cause of preventable, premature death in the United States. Worldwide. it is well documented that smoking causes heart disease, stroke, cancer, chronic obstructive lung disease, numerous diseases of the oral cavity, and complications during and after pregnancy.

There has also been a significant incidence in the use of smokeless tobacco by young males. Tobacco use is both dangerous and costly to our society. Smoking-attributable health care costs are estimated to be in excess of 300 billion dollars a year. This includes nearly 170 billion dollars for direct health care costs, 156 billion dollars for the cost of lost productivity and 5.6 billion dollars in loss of productivity caused by second hand exposure.. It is estimated that during their lifetime, female smokers will generate over $14,000 in additional medical costs and male smokers over $12,000 in additional medical costs.

Despite the devastating health consequences and staggering health care costs, clinicians often fail to assess and treat tobacco users consistently and effectively. This failure to assess and intervene with tobacco users occurs even though there is substantial evidence that brief interventions with tobacco users by medical and dental healthcare teams can be effective. In fact, 70% of adult tobacco users report that they would like to quit and would welcome advice from their health care providers.

TOBACCO PRODUCTS

Tobacco products should be considered chemically contaminated (toxic) nicotine delivery devices. Inhalation is not necessary for nicotine to be absorbed in the bloodstream. The pharmacologic objective of any tobacco form is the delivery of nicotine to the user's brain. Tobacco initiation and progression to nicotine addiction are influenced by sociocultural, psychological, physiologic, and genetic factors. Chronic tobacco use is characterized by psychological (habituation, behavioral) and pharmacologic (addiction, chemical dependency) factors. Table 1-2 provides an overview of the tobacco products consumed in the United States and lists the forms of tobacco products currently available. (See Figures 1-1 to 1-3).

Table 1 -2: Tobacco Products	
Pyrolytic (Combustion)	**Nonpyrolytic (Unburned)**
Cigarettes (95% of US tobacco consumed) Cigars Pipes	Smokeless (spit) (topical) tobacco Chewing tobacco, i.e., *Redman* Moist snuff, i.e., *Copenahgen*, *Skoal* Dry snuff (powdered)

The FDA recognizes tobacco in the following forms:
- Cigarettes
- Cigars, Little Cigars, Cigarillos
- Dissolvable Products
- Electronic Cigarettes (also referred to as: Vape Pen, e-Hookah, Hookah Pen)
- Traditional Smokeless Tobacco Products, Snus

- Waterpipes (also Referred to as: Hookah, Shisha, Narghile, Argileh)

CIGARETTE SMOKING

Cigarettes were first developed in the 1800s using "flu-cured" tobacco leaf, making it easier to inhale. Cigarettes consist of ground processed tobacco rolled in a flame-retardant paper. A filter is usually added. All tobacco forms contain tobacco toxins and carcinogens. The morbidity and mortality from chronic cigarette smoking are closely related to:
- Total years of smoking
- Number of cigarettes (packs) per day (pack-years-refers to the number of packs smoked per day times the number of years smoking)
- Depth of inhalation
- Use of filtered versus nonfiltered cigarettes
- Use of mentholated cigarette brands

The physicochemical nature of tobacco smoke is the result of:
- Pyrolysis (chemical decomposition of a substance by heat)
- Pyrosynthesis, and distillation during burning, which takes place within the pyrolytic cone found at the tip of the cigarette or cigar

Tobacco smoke is the visible vapor and gases given off during pyrolysis:
- Mainstream: smoke inhaled by the smoker
- Side stream: smoke emitted between puffs, also called secondary smoke

Environmental tobacco smoke is the sum total of all smoke produced. Carcinogenic substances found in tobacco smoke include:

As many as 7,200, chemical have been found in tobacco smoke. At least 45 chemicals found in tobacco smoke are classified as carcinogens.

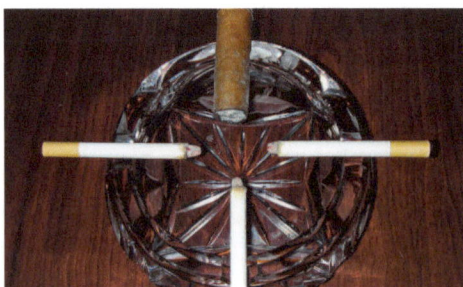

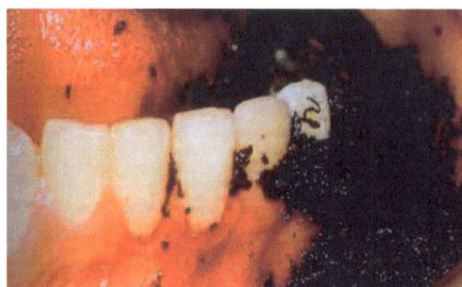

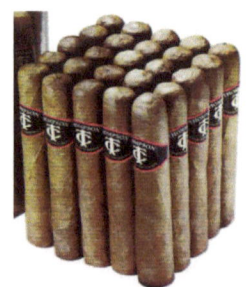

FIGURE 1-1: *Tobacco products consumed in the United States. A – Smoker's tobacco. B – Smokeless tobacco. C – Cigars*

Chemical components include:
- Carbon Monoxide
- Ammonia
- Acetylene
- Nicotine
- Cyanide
- Benzene
- Formaldehyde
- Tar
- Cadmium,
- Aromatic hydrocarbons
- Tobacco-specific N-nitrosamines
- Radioactive Polonium 210

Tobacco Chemical Toxicity

In 2012, for the first time, U.S. tobacco companies were required to report to the Food and Drug Administration (FDA) a list of chemicals and their amount that were in currently regulated tobacco products and tobacco smoke. These are chemicals or chemical compounds — that FDA calls Harmful and Potentially Harmful Constituents (HPHCs) — that cause, or could cause, harm to tobacco users or non-users. They have been found in cigarette smoke, cigarette filler, roll-your-own tobacco and smokeless tobacco. Different tobacco products may contain different HPHCs, and some HPHCs are created when the chemicals are burned.

FDA's Center for Tobacco Products (CTP) has established an initial list of 93 HPHCs, and has identified a shortened list of 20 chemicals. This action is required by the Family Smoking Prevention and Tobacco Control Act that was passed by Congress and signed by President Obama in 2009. The law requires tobacco companies to report this information to FDA, and FDA is required to inform the public about the quantity of chemicals that may cause disease in specific tobacco products, and the adverse effects.

The FDA reports there are more than 7,000 chemicals in tobacco and tobacco smoke. A list of 93 HPHCs included on the list have been identified as causes or possible causes of cancer, cardiovascular disease, respiratory effects, developmental or reproductive effects, and addiction to tobacco products.

CIGAR SMOKING

In 2014 approximately 13 billion cigars were sold in the United States. A cigar is any roll of tobacco wrapped in leaf tobacco or in any substance containing tobacco. A single cigar may contain more tobacco than one or two packages of cigarettes. The average cigarette is smoked for 7 minutes using 10 puffs. Because of size, a typical cigar is consumed with 100 puffs over a considerably longer period of time. One cigar in a 30-minute period can produce the equivalent environmental tobacco smoke of 42 cigarettes.

Concerns
- Systemic and upper aerodigestive tract disease consequences
- Risk of nicotine addiction
- Environmental cigar smoke significantly contributes to indoor air pollution
- Adolescent use, "blunting": cigars used as an illicit drug delivery system
- Since 1993, in the United States, cigar sales have increased by 50%. Increased use rates are noted in adults, females, and adolescents.
- The dose-response relationship for excess disease risk depends on the number of cigars smoked daily, the depth of inhalation and the number of years of use.

Types of Cigars
- Little (<3 lb/1,000) (1.3 – 2.5 g weight, 70-120 mm length)
- Small (cigarillos)
- Regular (>3 lb/1,000) (5 – 17 g weight, 110-150 mm length, 17 mm diameter)
- Premium (very large, hand rolled, costly) (22 g weight, 127 – 124 mm length, 12 – 23 mm diameter)

Cigar Smoke
- Cigar smoke has the same toxic and carcinogenic compounds identified in cigarette smoke.
- Cigar smoking is not a safe alternative to cigarette smoking.
- Unburned cigars expose the lips and oral cavity to topical tobacco toxins and carcinogens.
- The risk of oral and oropharyngeal cancers is similar to that of cigarette smokers; the overall risk is 7 to 10 times greater than that of never-smokers.
- Moderate inhalation of five cigars daily creates lung cancer risk equal to smoking one pack per day.
- Nicotine in cigar smoke is readily absorbed across the upper digestive tract mucosa in addition to being absorbed during pulmonary inhalation.

PIPE SMOKING

Pipe smoking poses health risks that are similar to those associated with cigar smoking. Environmental tobacco smoke from pipe smoking creates indoor air pollution and is a health risk to nonsmokers. The thermal effects of the pipe stem and the hot gases produced during combustion act synergistically with the toxic components in pipe tobacco smoke. This enhances the risk of carcinogenesis in those chronically exposed tissues, such as the lips and the oral soft palate.

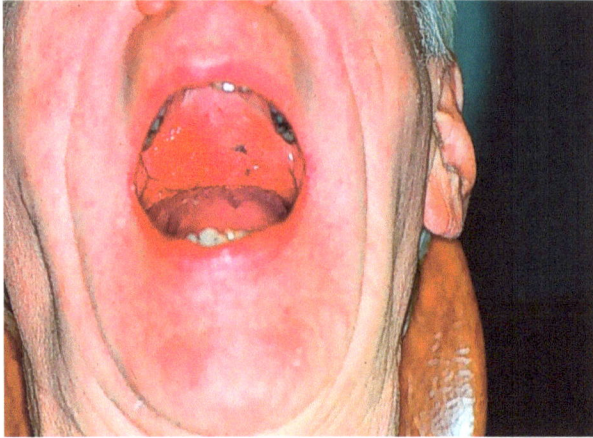

FIGURE 1-2: *Soft plate squamous cell cancer Stage II at the location of pipe stem placement in chronic pipe smoker*

SMOKELESS (SPIT, TOPICAL) TOBACCO

Approximately 128 million pounds of smokeless tobacco was sold in the united states in 2013 up from 125.5 million pounds the year before. The intraorally placed bolus of salivated tobacco is called a "quid." In 1986, the US Surgeon General's Report on smokeless tobacco determined that "...the oral use of smokeless tobacco represents a significant health risk. It is not a safe substitute for cigarette smoking. It can cause cancer and a number of non-cancerous oral conditions and lead to nicotine addiction and dependence." In 2015, the CDC reported that high school athletes were more likely to use smokeless tobacco products than non-athletes.

There are two types of smokeless tobacco with over 90% sold by three companies (American Snuff, Swedish Match and U.S. Smokeless Tobacco Company):

- Chewing tobacco (three forms)
  - Loose leaf (shredded)
  - Plugs (pressed into bricks)
  - Twists (dried and twisted into rope-like strands)

- Snuff: powered or finely cut cured tobacco leaves (two forms)
  - Moist
  - Dry powdered

There is compelling evidence that smokeless tobacco is dangerous and highly addictive. Manufacturers

chemically alter the pH of these products by adding alkaline buffering agents. This enhances the efficacy of trans-mucosal absorption into the bloodstream when it is placed in the buccal vestibule. Sustained high-frequency spit tobacco use has been associated with many adverse oral and dental conditions.

In addition to the commonly used products, such as cigarettes, chew dip, pipes, and cigars, several "new" tobacco products have been marketed and these should be considered equally as dangerous and not safe alternatives to smoking. These products are known as bidis, herbal cigarettes, low-nicotine cigarettes (*Omni*), and tobacco lozenges (*Arriva* lozenges, not to be confused with *Commit* nicotine lozenges). A brief description follows.

Bidis are hand-rolled cigarettes consisting of ground tobacco rolled in a tobacco or tendu leaf with flavoring added. This product is primarily made in India using child labor. They are very strong and produce up to three times as much nicotine and five times as much tar as regular cigarettes. These products are sold via the black market and can be found in some stores that sell drug paraphernalia, often called "head shops."

Herbal cigarettes are usually some type of herb that is often ground up with tobacco (to aid in slow burning). They produce tars and carbon monoxide. Young people often consider these cigarettes as "better for their health" because they contain herbs.

Omni cigarettes are marketed by the tobacco industry as less addicting because they have low nicotine delivery. They produce tar and carbon monoxide similar to that of regular cigarettes.

Arriva tobacco lozenges are produced by the tobacco industry. This product contains finely ground tobacco in a candy coating. They likely carry the same risks as smokeless tobacco and are likely to be carcinogenic.

SNUS

A new addition to the tobacco product market are Snus, These flavored pouches are finely ground moist snuff in a teabag-like pouch that are placed in the oral mucosal vestibule. These products are not messy and can clandestinely deliver significant levels of nicotine without any combustion products. They are manufactured to have lower level of TSNAS, The safety and adverse health effects of snus are being studied.

ELECTRONIC NICOTINE DELIVERY SYSTEMS

Electronic cigarettes, also known as e-cigarettes, are battery-operated products designed to deliver nicotine, flavor and other chemicals. They turn chemicals, including highly addictive nicotine, into an aerosol that is inhaled by the user. Most e-cigarettes are manufactured to look like conventional cigarettes, cigars, or pipes. Some resemble everyday items such as pens and USB memory sticks for people who wish to use the product without others noticing. The devices are intended for user nicotine delivery and behavioral appeasement. A single puff from an e-cigarette may deliver about 10% of the nicotine as puff from a conventional cigarette. Users refer to use as "vaping."

Electronic cigarettes deliver nicotine or other substances to a user in the form of a vapor. Typically, they are composed of a rechargeable, battery-operated heating element, a replaceable cartridge that may contain nicotine or other chemicals, and an atomizer that, when heated, converts the contents of the cartridge into a vapor. This vapor can then be inhaled by the user and the nicotine absorbed in the same manner as cigarette smoking.

E-cigarettes have not been fully studied and the FDA has not evaluated any e-cigarette products for safety or effectiveness. The FDA found significant issues that indicate that quality control processes used to manufacture these products are substandard or non-existent. Concerns have been raised that the marketing of products such as e-cigarettes can increase nicotine addiction among young people may result in kids trying other tobacco products. Consumers may not know the potential risks of e-cigarettes when used as intended, how much nicotine or other potentially harmful chemicals are being inhaled during use, or whether there are any benefits associated with using these products.

In 2015, the FDA reported adverse events involving e-cigarettes from consumers, health professionals and concerned members of the public. The adverse events have included hospitalization for illnesses such as: pneumonia, congestive heart failure, disorientation, seizure and hypotension. Whether e-cigarettes caused these reported adverse events is unknown and more research is needed. One clinical anecdotal incidence reveals a spontaneous failure and explosion of an e-cigarette that caused considerable oro-facial trauma, including intra-oral burns, luxation injuries and alveolar fracture (Harrison, 2015).

The FDA is concerned about the safety of these products and how they are marketed to the public Concerns include:

- e-cigarettes can increase nicotine addiction among young people and may lead kids to try other tobacco products, including conventional cigarettes, which are known to cause disease and lead to premature death
- the products may contain ingredients that are known to be toxic to humans
- because clinical studies about the safety and efficacy of these products for their intended use have not been submitted to FDA, consumers currently have no way of knowing whether e-cigarettes are safe for their intended use or about what types or concentrations of potentially harmful chemicals or what dose of nicotine they are inhaling when they use these products.

It is appropriate that parents tell their children and teenagers that these products are not safe to use. Of particular concern to parents is that e-cigarettes may be sold without any legal age restrictions, and are available in different flavors (including chocolate, strawberry and mint) which may appeal to young people. Additionally, the devices do not contain any health warnings comparable to FDA-approved nicotine replacement products or conventional cigarettes.

In 2016 the National Institute on Drug Abuse stated that **teenagers are more likely to use e-cigarettes than cigarettes with twice as** many boys using e-cigarettes than girls. **Teen e-cig users are more likely to start smoking** combustible tobacco products (cigarettes, cigars, and hookahs) and **most teens are unaware of what substances are in their e-cigarette**. Additionally 7 in 10 middle school and high school teens are exposed to e-cig advertizing including retail, internet, television and movie ads and by newspaper and magazine advertisements. The U.S Surgeon General in 2016 stated that the use of e-cigarettes pose significant risk to younger users, likely impairing normal brain development.

When used as manufacturer directed e-cigarettes simulate the bio behavioral aspects (visual, sensory, manual) of smoking conventional combusted cigarette. Currently there are a variety brands and designs available including three categories: *cigalikes* (cigarette sized in shape and size), *egos* (larger than *cigalikes*, typically with a removable refillable e-liquid nicotine tank, and *mods* larger than *cigalikes* with the capacity to be customized to individual preference.

Adverse Oral Health Effects of e-Cigarettes:

Cigarette smoking and exposure to nicotine increase the incidence and severity of periodontal disease. As many as

4,700 chemicals are found in cigarette smoke including nicotine, oxidants and free radicals.

Nicotine is a vasoconstrictor and the effects are both topical and systemic. Neutrophil chemotaxis and phagocytotic capacity are reduced in smokers compared to non-smokers. Additionally, smokers comparatively have lower IgA, IgG, IgM and suppressor CD8 lymphocytes. These factors adversely affect localized immume and inflammatory response in periodontal disease. A number of proposed mechanisms have been implicated on the singular adverse affect of nicotine on periodontal health.

In addition to health concerns associated the vapor produced by electronic nicotine delivery systems concerns about safety have been noted. The user is directly exposed to the vapor as well as other individuals in the immediate vicinity. The lithium ion battery has been linked to unintentional fires as a result of manufacture defects and overcharging. The nicotine replacement cartridge contains a significant amount of potentially toxic nicotine, has resulted in incidents of pediatric poisoning. The delivery system cartridge may be tampered with and there is the possibility that it may be used to administer illicit drugs, especially in underage individuals. The vaporized aerosol contains water, nicotine, humectants, propylene glycol, glycerol and various flavorings agents. The adverse effect and the safety of some of these chemical constituents have yet to be confirmed. Some of the product cartridges are manufactured outside of the United States and the presence of contaminates, including lead and formaldehyde, has raised questions on quality assurance.

Tobacco Harm Reduction (THR)

Manufacturing promotion and advertisement have marketed e-cigarettes as another tobacco smoke-free alternative to nicotine delivery and as a tobacco cessation aid. Electronic nicotine delivery systems have been referred to as "tobacco harm reduction". Options for active tobacco users include quitting, continuing to use at current at reduced levels or using a harm reduction strategy. It has been proposed that a harm reduction approach may significantly reduce the morbidity and premature mortality associated with cigarette smoking. At the time of this monogram publication the actual health effects to users and others, the safety, social acceptability and the effectiveness as a tobacco substitute are not known. As of 2016 the FDA has ruled that e-cigarettes may not be marketed as safe alternatives to cigarettes or as a smoking cessation product and must be sold as smokeless tobacco products.

Conclusion:

Although there are many unknowns regarding the health and safety of e-cigarette use their popularity is on the increase. The health risk is likely to be similar to smokeless tobacco, which has approximately 1% of the mortality of smoking cigarettes. Issues of safeguarding public health and formulating regulatory strategies include product design and safety, toxicant exposure to user and bystanders, youth initiation and as a tobacco cessation method. At the time of this monogram publication the use of electronic nicotine delivery systems are assessed as not a safe alternative to cigarettes or as an approved smoking cessation product.

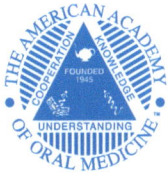

2   Tobacco Use and Oral Diseases

MUCOSAL CONDITIONS

Oral Cancer (Squamous Cell Carcinoma)

Oral cancer accounts for 4% of all cancers. In the U.S., up to 50,000 new cases of oral cancer are diagnosed every year and the annual mortality rate is approaching 10,000 people. The median 5-year survival rate is 64%. Approximately 8 out of 10 patients diagnosed with oral cancer are current smokers and the incidence of oral cancer among smokers varies from 2-18 times that of non-smokers. The greatest risk is tobacco users who regularly use alcohol due to an enhanced synergistic effect; the use of both account for approximately 75% of all oral and oropharyngeal cancers in the US. Ninety-five percent of all oral cancer occur in persons older than 40 years, with the male to female ratio being 2:1. In smokers and drinkers, it is estimated that 97% of the oral cancers will occur on the floor of the mouth, ventrolateral surface of the tongue, and soft palate complex.

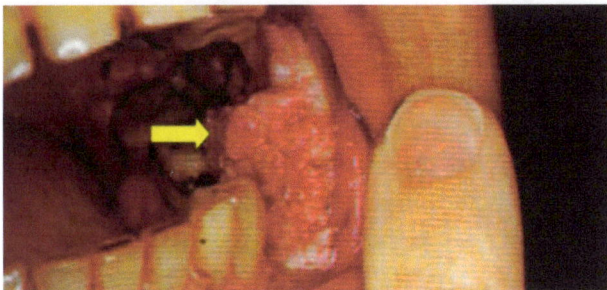

FIGURE 2–1: *Squamous cell carcinoma of the left buccal mucosa and vestibule of a chronic smoker*

Leukoplakia

Leukoplakia is a white plaque of questionable risk having excluded other known disorders or diseases that carry no increased risk for cancer. Leukoplakia occurs six times more frequently in smokers than in non-smokers. Leukoplakia is a clinical descriptive term and refers to a partially or completely demarcated white plaque that usually exhibts internal fissuring. Non-homogenous leukoplakias (eg. erythroleukoplakia, speckled leukoplakia) have a higher malignant potential risk. Histologic examination is required to rule out dysplasia and even cases with no dysplasia (keratosis of unknown significance) must be followed closely (see Figures 2-2 & 2-3).

FIGURE 2–2: A – *Leukoplakia of the left buccal mucosa in a chronic tobacco user.*
B – *A burn from smoking unfiltered cigarettes on the lower labial mucosa.*
C – *Homgenous leukoplakia on the right posterior mandibular facial alveolar mucosa. Note the heavy nicotine staining on teeth.*
D – *Speckled leukoplakia on the labial mucosa and labial vestibule due to use of smokeless tobacco.*

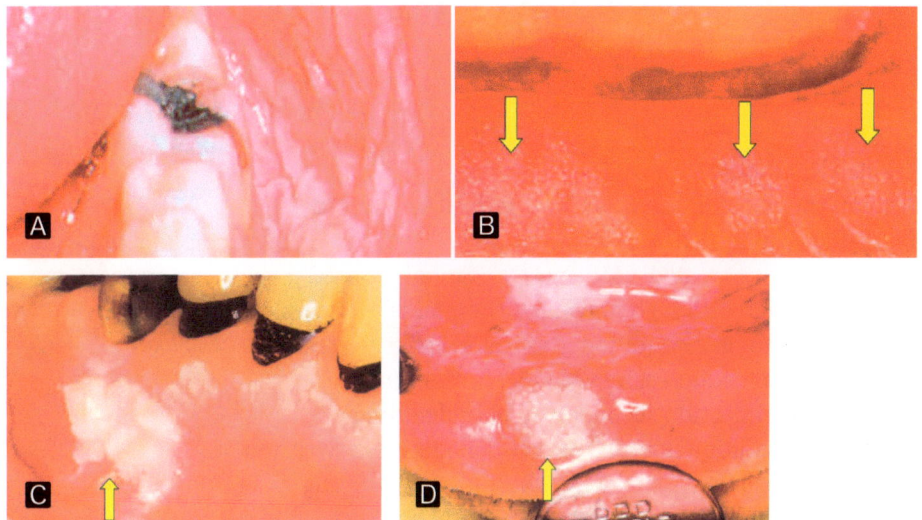

FIGURE 2–3: *A – Nodular non-homogenous leukoplakia of the hard palate in a chronic smoker.*
B – Verrucous carcinoma of the right mandibular vestibule/labial mucosa in a tobacco chewer.
C – Speckled leukoplakia of the left buccal mucosa.
D – Speckled leukoplakia of the left anterior buccal mucosa and commissure.

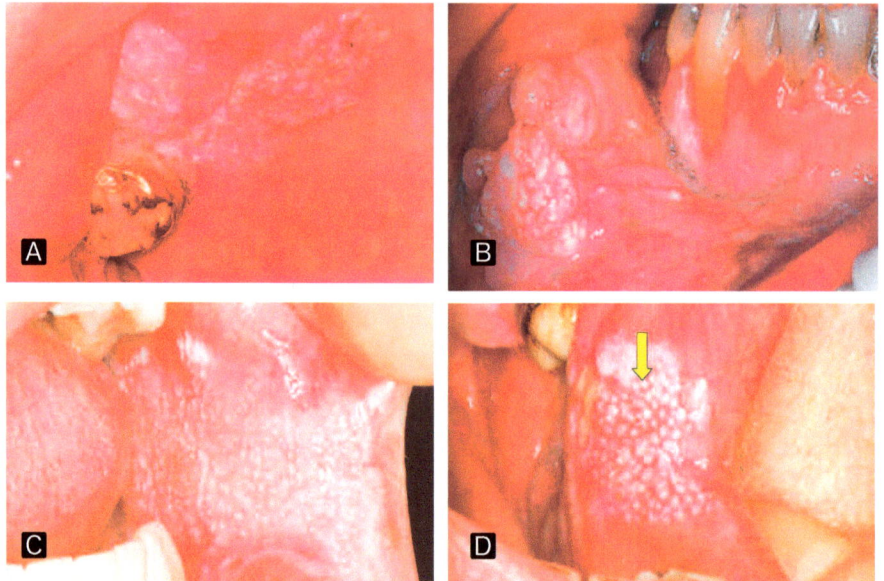

Chronic Hyperplastic Candidiasis

Chronic hyperplastic candidiasis presents as a leukoplakia or erythroleukoplakia that cannot be wiped away and is most commonly seen on the anterior buccal mucosae (see Figure 2-4). This lesion is characterized by the presence of candida hyphae on histopathologic examination and may or may not feature dysplasia. This lesion is usually seen in chronic smokers and carries a significant malignant potential. At this time, it is unknown if certain pathogenic strains of Candida Albicans induce dysplasia or if the lesion creates an enivirment for secondary candidal colonization. Occassionaly lesions regress with anti-fungal therapy.

FIGURE 2–4:
Chronic hyperplastic candidiasis of the anterior buccal mucosa of a chronic smoker

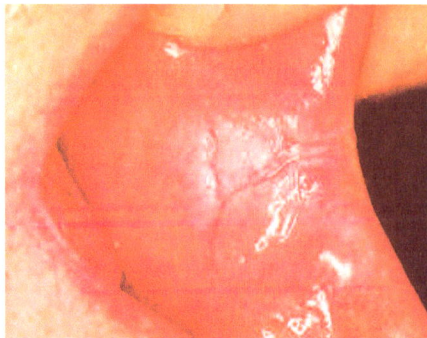

Median Rhomboid Glossitis

Median rhomboid glossitis is characterized by a well-demarcated symmetrical erythematous patch devoid of filiform papillae located on the posterior midline of the tongue dorsum. Although previously thought to be a developmental tongue condition, this lesion is likely a result of local immunosuppressive therapies, chronic smoking, and candidal infection secondary to poor denture hygiene. The condition is usually asymptomatic however if symptoms arise (mainly burning), initiation of antifungal therapy is appropriate.

Nicotine Stomatitis

Nicotine stomatitis develops in response to heat generated from cigar and pipe smoking and less frequently from cigarette smoking. Long-term heat exposure results in diffuse palatal hyperkeratosis (see Figure 2-5). Squamous metaplasia of the minor salivary gland ducts results in multiple punctate red papules on a background of diffuse white palatal hyperkeratosis (see Figure 2-6). This condition does not carry a malignant transformation potential and if the smoking habit is ceased, normal mucosa will return in approximately two weeks.

FIGURE 2–5:
Nicotine stomatitis on the palate of a pipe smoker

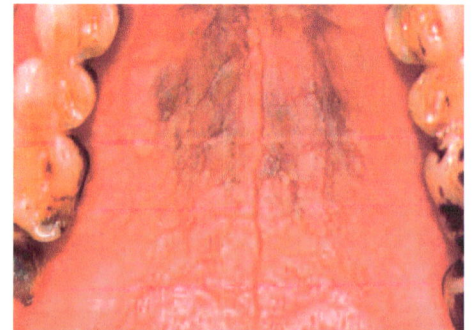

FIGURE 2–6:
Palatal nicotine stomatitis in a chronic cigar smoker

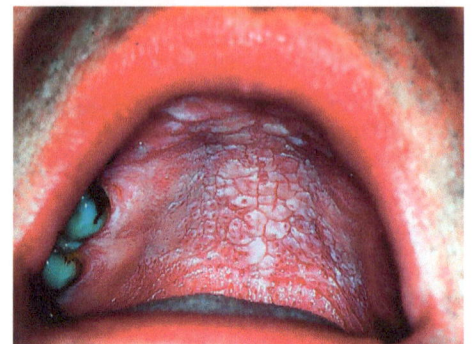

Smokeless tobacco keratosis

Tobacco chewing, dry snuff and moist snuff are the main types of smokeless tobacco consumed in the US. Approximately 3% of the US population consume smokeless tobacco products. Commercial smokeless tobacco products contain many tobacco-specific N-nitrosamines that have been implicated as carcinogens known to disrupt DNA repair. Clinically this lesion features a whitish gray plaque with internal fissuring and parallel ridging in the area in direct contact to the smokeless tobacco. The lesion usually develops after at least one year of smokeless tobacco consumption and will regress when tobacco use is completely discontinued (see Figure 2-7). A recent systematic review and meta-analysis determined that snuff consumption is strongly associated with the risk of oral cancer (OR = 3.01).

Smoker's Melanosis

Tobacco smoke stimulates basal melanocytes to produce melanin and diffuse oral pigmentation may result. Brownish black pigmentation sometimes with a yellow hue is often seen on the facial attached gingiva. The intensity of pigmentation seen in smoker's melanosis is time and dose dependent and is reversible with smoking cessation.

Black Hairy Tongue

Hairy tongue arises from the overgrowth of filiform papillae and from retention keratosis. Several factors including chronic smoking, salivary hypofuction, poor oral and tongue hygiene provide and environment for chromogenic bacteria to induce black hairy tongue (see Figure 2-8). Cessation of smoking and adequate tongue brushing will reverse this condition.

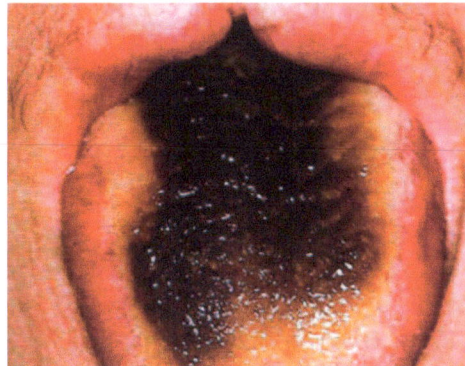

FIGURE 2–8: *Black hairy tongue of a tobacco smoker*

DENTAL CONDITIONS

Staining of Teeth and Restorative Materials

Tobacco users experience increased rates (~67%) of tooth loss compared to non-smokers. Tobacco stains can adhere and penetrate into enamel, dentin and cementum, and resin-based restorative materials, creating brown to yellow discoloration of these surfaces. Dentures and other prosthetic appliances may also be stained by repeated exposure to tobacco.

Abrasion

Excessive pipe smoking has a considerable abrasive potential and may result in significant tooth abrasion, producing

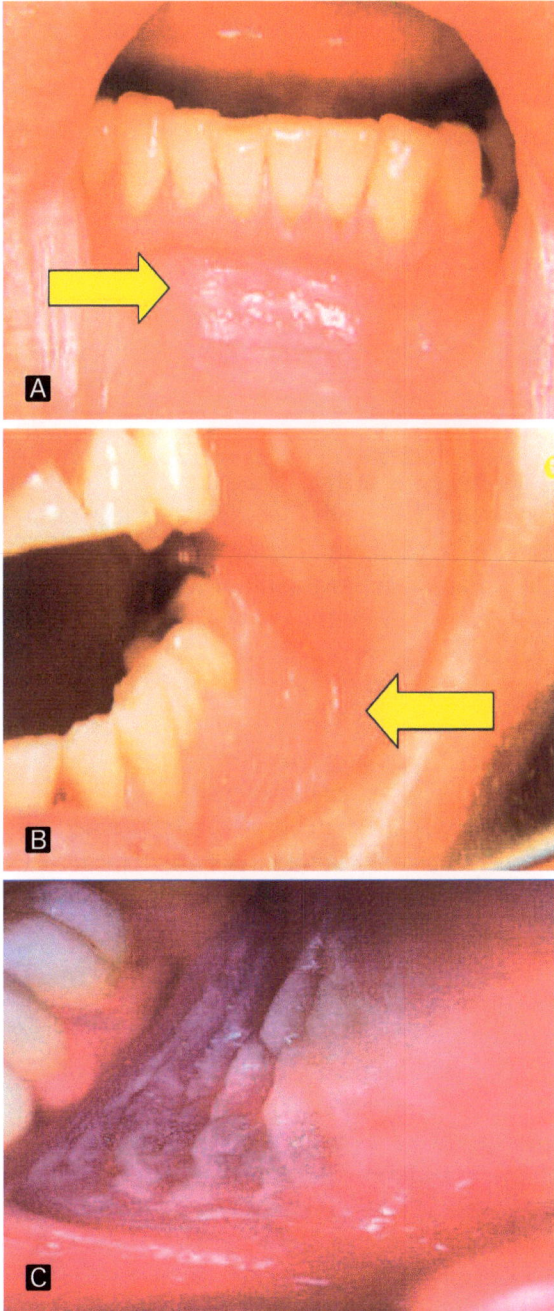

FIGURE 2–7: *A, B, C – Snuff dipper's pouch formation in the mouths of snuff users*

notches or wear patterns along occlusal surfaces. Abrasives in chewing tobacco may also wear away a considerable portion of the surfaces of teeth contacting the tobacco.

Dental Caries

The incidence of dental caries may be greater in smokers than in non-smokers. However, some researchers have suggested that the abrasive action, fluoride content, and increased salivary flow in chewing tobacco may decrease caries activity. Researchers have analyzed dental caries and tobacco use data from more than 14,000 individuals aged 18 years and older (between 1988 and 1994). Survey data revealed that 6% of men aged 18 years and older use some form of spit tobacco. Almost half of those men who use chewing tobacco also have one or more decayed or filled root surfaces. Men who used chewing tobacco exclusively had 3.84 decayed or filled root surfaces (of 112 possible surfaces), more than any other tobacco use group and those who had never used tobacco. The more packages of chewing tobacco that a man used each week, the more likely he was to have a decayed or filled root surface. The more years that a man had used chewing tobacco, the more likely he was to have a decayed or filled root surface. Researchers speculate that the high sugar content in some chewing tobacco products is one reason that the product is associated with an increased risk of dental caries on coronal and root surfaces.

PERIODONTAL CONDITIONS

Smoking is a major risk factor for periodontal disease. Both current and former smokers have an increased prevalence and severity of periodontal disease. There is a significant dose-dependent relationship between the amount of smoked cigarettes and the severity of periodontitis. Smokers in general have a 4 to 6 times greater risk of periodontitis than non-smokers when all other risk factors are adjusted for.

Cigarette smoking and exposure to nicotine increase the incidence and severity of periodontal disease. As many as 4,700 chemicals are found in cigarette smoke including nicotine, oxidants and free radicals. Nicotine is a vasoconstrictor and the effects are both topical and systemic. Neutrophil chemotaxis and phagocytotic capacity are reduced in smokers compared to non-smokers. Additionally, smokers comparatively have lower IgA, IgG, IgM and suppressor CD8 lymphocytes. These factors adversely affect localized immune and inflammatory response in periodontal disease. A number of proposed mechanisms have been implicated on the singular adverse affect of nicotine on periodontal health.

Smoking-Associated Periodontitis

Fibrotic gingiva with thickened rolled margins appear in smokers. Minimal gingival redness or edema, greater pocketing in anterior and palatal sites, and recession in anterior segments are also found. Clinical characteristics of periodontitis among smokers include early onset of disease at ages 20 to 30, relatively rapid disease progression, and minimal reduction in gingival pocket depth following scaling.

Acute Necrotizing Ulcerative Gingivitis

This condition clinically presents with punched-out interdental papillae and gingival tissues that bleed easily. The mouth is painful and presents a distinctive fetid odor. Poor oral hygiene, tobacco use, emotional stress, and decreased circulation contribute to the causation of this disease.

Gingival Recession

Smokeless tobacco use increases the risk of localized gingival recession. The gingiva tends to be more fibrotic, with thickened rolled margins in smokers. Gingival recession usually occurs in areas in direct contact with the smokeless tobacco.

Plaque and Calculus Formation

Plaque and calculus buildup are accelerated in smokers. Impairment of the local immune system, including reduction in salivary immunoglobulin A secretion and a reduction in salivary flow rates are contributory factors in smokers.

ORAL HYGIENE

Reduced taste and smell acuity may produce dietary changes, such as the increased dietary use of salt, sugar, and spices. Halitosis is one of the most commonly recognized conditions associated with tobacco use. If tobacco use is discontinued and overall oral hygiene is improved, this condition will likely regress.

Effects on Diagnosis, Prognosis, and Therapy

Impaired healing and poorer clinical results following both non-surgical and surgical periodontal therapy of smokers versus non-smokers is a common challenge experienced by smokers. Additionally, less reduction in bleeding on probing and smaller gain in attachment may become problematic. Soft tissue and bone graft procedures are less successful in smokers versus non-smokers. Guided tissue regeneration procedures tend to be less successful in addition.

Implants

Dental implant failure in smokers is significantly higher than in non-smokers. Impaired wound healing is a result of vasoconstriction and increased platelet aggregation (decreased blood flow). Increased levels of carboxyhemoglobin (decreased oxygen transport), changes in vascular endothelium, and elevated levels of tumor necrosis factor α in the gingival crevicular fluid are frequently seen in smokers.

Delayed Wound Healing

Smoking cessation should be considered an integral part of periodontal treatment. Vasoconstriction of blood vessels contributes significantly to delaying wound healing.

Dry Socket (Acute Alveolar Osteitis)

The ischemic effect of tobacco use and impairment of the immune system may lead to increased incidence of dry sockets (post-extraction acute alveolar osteitis) among smokers. The risk of post-extraction acute alveolar osteitis is significantly lessened if the patient is instructed to cease smoking for as long as possible following the dental extraction(s).

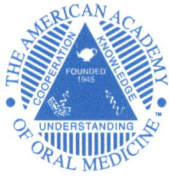

3 Tobacco Use and Systemic Diseases

There is no safe from of tobacco; all tobacco products contain nicotine and carcinogens which have adverse systemic and oral health consequences. (Bertazzo-Silveira) (Munshi), In the US, the risk of mortality from cigarette smoking has increased for both genders in the last 50 years. Currently, cigarette smoking is the leading preventable cause of mortality in the US with approximately 480,000 deaths annually. Cigarette smoking accounts for approximately 1 in 5 deaths in the US.

CARDIOVASCULAR DISEASE

The link between coronary heart disease and smoking was first reported in 1940. Since then, the association between cigarette smoking and an increased risk of stroke, myocardial infarction, peripheral vascular disease, aortic aneurysm, and sudden death has been well documented. Chronic cigarette smoking is estimated to increase the risk of both stroke and coronary heart disease by two to four times that of non-smokers. Atherosclerotic peripheral artery disease affects 8.5 million people in the US. Atherosclerotic peripheral artery disease is highly associated with adverse cardiovascular events and related mortality. Smoking and diabetes are the strongest risk factors for atherosclerotic peripheral artery disease. Smoking cessation significantly reduces the risk of adverse cardiovascular events and related mortality compared to those who continue to smoke.

Cigarette smoke causes damage to vascular endothelium, which results in the initiation of atherosclerosis. Coronary artery vaso-occlusive factors include increased platelet aggregation, increased vasomotor reactivity, increased prothrombotic state, increased fibrinogen levels, increased carbon monoxide, increased plasma viscosity, increased risk of coronary artery vasospasm and elevated total cholesterol, and decreased high-density lipoprotein. Smokers with coronary heart disease may have 33% more episodes of ischemia per day, and these episodes are likely to be of longer duration than those of nonsmokers. There is also an increased risk of ventricular fibrillation and cardiac arrest.

LUNG DISEASES

Cigarette smoking is the leading cause of pulmonary diseases in the United States. Chronic obstructive pulmonary disease (COPD) is the third leading cause of death in the United States today. Over 11 million Americans suffer from COPD today with millions more living with the disease that are undiagnosed.

COPD is an irreversible obstructive airflow of the lungs. The two most common disorders classified as COPD are bronchitis and emphysema. Cigarette smoking accounts for approximately 80% of COPD mortality in both males and females. Male smokers have an eight-fold increased risk and female smokers have a six-fold greater risk of COPD than non-smokers. It is estimated that male and female smokers are 12-13 times more likely to die from COPD than non-smokers.

Bronchitis is characterized by increased mucus production in the tracheobronchial tissues, which often results in a chronic cough with expectoration. Recurrent infections with *Streptococcus pneumoniae* and *Haemophilus influenzae* are common. The pathophysiology of bronchitis includes thickened bronchial walls with an inflammatory infiltrate, an increase in the size of the mucous glands, goblet cell hyperplasia, narrowing of the small airways, mucous plugging, collapse of the peripheral airways owing to loss of surfactant, and obstruction of airflow on both inspiration and expiration.

Emphysema is characterized by distention of the air spaces distal to the terminal bronchioles and the destruction of the alveolar septa. The pathophysiology of emphysema includes enlargement of the air spaces distal to the terminal bronchioles, destruction of the alveolar walls and loss of elastic recoil of the lung. Obstruction results from the collapse of the enlarged air spaces on expiration.

CANCER

Oral Cancer

Tobacco accounts for at least 93% of cancers of the oral cavity and oropharynx in males and 61% of oral and oropharyngeal cancers in females. Approximately 8 out of 10 patients diagnosed with oral cancer are current smokers and the incidence of oral cancer among smokers varies from 2-18 times that of non-smokers. Cigarette smokers have a 5-9 fold increased risk of oral cancer compared to non-smokers, and this risk is dose-dependent and increases directly with the number of cigarettes smoked and the duration of smoking. Cigarettes, cigars, pipes, and smokeless tobacco can cause oral cancer. The greatest risk is tobacco users who regularly use alcohol due to an enhanced synergistic effect; the use of both account for approximately 75% of all oral and oropharyngeal cancers in the US. In the US, up to 50,000 new cases of oral cancer are diagnosed every year and the annual mortality rate is approaching 10,000 people. The cancer risk increase may be as much as 17 times greater for smokers consuming greater than 80 cigarettes per day.

Cigarette smokers who have been diagnosed with an oral cancer are at increased risk of the development of other primary malignancies. Oral cancer patients who have undergone therapy and continue to smoke have a 2-6 times greater risk of a second malignancy in the aerodigestive tract. The carcinogens found in mainstream tobacco smoke are tobacco-specific N-nitrosamines, aromatic amines, and polycyclic aromatic hydrocarbons and Polonium 210. The annual incidence of oropharyngeal cancer is 12.4 in 100,000 for blacks and 9.7 in 100,000 for whites. The highest rate is 20.5 in 100,000 for black males. Over 90% of oral cancers occur in individuals over the age of 45 years. There is a 2:1 male to female ratio; however, this ratio has become less dramatic over the past 40 years because more women have been exposing themselves to tobacco. It is estimated that 97% of the oral cancers will occur on the floor of the mouth, ventrolateral surface of the tongue, and soft palate complex. The median 5-year survival rate is 64%, with a mortality rate of 2.4 in 100,000 for whites and 4.4 in 100,000 for blacks. The 5-year survival is directly dependent on the stage of the cancer at the time of diagnosis.

The diagnosis of obvious and advanced oral squamous cell carcinoma may not be clinically very difficult. The challenge is in the early diagnosis of asymptomatic squamous cell carcinoma. To improve the survival of the oral cancer patient, the oral health care provider must perform a thorough intraoral examination (oral cancer screening examination), determine the patient's risk factors for oral cancer, and be aware of the clinical characteristics of early, asymptomatic oral cancer.

Lung Cancer

Prior to the twentieth century, lung cancer was a rare disease. Lung cancer death rates began to rise among males in the 1930s, which was more than 20 years after the increase in smoking among males. Changes in the cigarette-related mortality risk for lung cancer between Cancer Prevention Study I and Cancer Prevention Study II revealed that for males, the relative risk of lung cancer had increased from 11.9 to 23.2. This was reflected by an increase from 91.6 to 95.7% in the percentage of deaths attributed to lung cancer. For females, the relative risk increased from 2.7 to 12.8 and the percentage of deaths attributed to lung cancer increased from 63.4 to 92.2%. In 2005, the number of lung cancer deaths peaked to the highest recorded levels of 159,292 but has fortunately decreased to 155,610 in 2014. However, an estimated 158,080 people will succumb to lung cancer this year.

Today, cigarette smoking accounts for approximately 90% of all lung cancer deaths. Lung cancer is the leading cause of cancer death in the US (~27% of all cancer deaths) for both genders and has surpassed breast cancer in women as the leading cause of death. There is a significant difference in smoking associated lung cancer incidence and mortality among men and women. Compared to non-smokers, male current smokers are ~23 times more likely to develop lung cancer and women are ~13 times more likely to develop lung cancer. Men have a higher risk of dying from lung cancer than women. The rates of lung cancer have increased over the past 60 years, and this increase is directly related to the number of cigarettes smoked. An Environmental Protection Agency study estimated that environmental tobacco smoke (second-hand smoke) is responsible for 3,000 deaths every year. Another study estimated that 17% of cases of lung cancer in non-smokers may be attributed to exposure to high levels of tobacco smoke during childhood years.

Other Cancers

In addition to oral cancer and lung cancer, cigarette use is strongly linked to cancers of the esophagus, stomach, pancreas, uterus, cervix, kidney, urethra, bladder, and myeloid leukemia. Compared to non-smokers, esophageal cancer risk is 3-7 times greater in current smokers. There is a dose-dependent relationship between the number of cigarettes smoked per day and the duration of smoking with the risk of esophageal cancer. Furthermore, worse survival outcomes are seen in heavy tobacco users. There is an approximate 70% synergistic risk reduction of esophageal cancer with combined smoking and alcohol cessation. When compared with non-smokers, there is a threefold increase in the risk of cutaneous squamous cell carcinoma in smokers. Current or past smokers have an increased risk of impotency after radiation therapy for prostate cancer. Smoking can cause colon cancer and causes microsatellite instability in colonic tumors. Smoking increases the risk of colorectal cancer death and the risk of gastrointestinal complications after radiation therapy for cervical cancer.

Gastrointestinal Diseases
Smokers have an increased risk of peptic ulcer disease and an increased risk of Crohn's disease that has an associated poorer prognosis.

Arthritis
Smokers have an increased risk of rheumatoid arthritis.

Ocular Diseases
Smokers have an increased risk of cataracts and an increased risk of age-related macular degeneration.

Depression
Smokers are more likely to be depressed and have a higher prevalence of anxiety disorders, bulimia, attention-deficit disorder, alcohol abuse, and schizophrenia.

Endocrine Diseases
Smokers have an increased risk of Graves' exophthalmia. Smoking affects glucose regulation. Smokers have an increased risk of dysmenorrhea and menstrual irregularity. Smokers experience natural menopause at a younger age and are more likely to experience menopausal symptoms.

Reproductive System
Smokers have an increased risk of infertility, ectopic pregnancies and spontaneous abortions. Complications caused by smoking during pregnancy include pre-term delivery, abruptio placentae, and placenta previa. Perinatal mortality increases in smokers, causing still-birth, neonatal death, and an increased rate of sudden infant death syndrome. Infants born to smoking mothers have a lower birth weight.

Bone Density
Postmenopausal women who smoke have a lower bone density and an increased risk of hip fracture.

ENVIRONMENTAL TOBACCO SMOKE (Second-Hand Smoke)
In June 2002, the International Agency for Research on Cancer stated that involuntary smoking (second-hand smoke) is carcinogenic to humans. Exposure to second-hand smoke is particularly damaging to the lungs of infants. Second-hand smoke is associated with an increased risk of bronchitis and pneumonia in children. It is also associated with an increase in the number of new cases of asthma in children, increased frequency of asthmatic episodes, and increased severity of asthmatic attacks. In-utero exposure to second-hand smoke results in decreased lung function in infants and decreased pulmonary functional activity in adolescence. Every year, 3,000 lung cancer deaths and 62,000 deaths from coronary heart disease in adult non-smokers are attributed to second-hand smoke. Two health objectives for Healthy People 2010 are to reduce cigarette smoking among adults to 12% and to reduce the proportion of non-smokers exposed to environmental smoke to 45%.

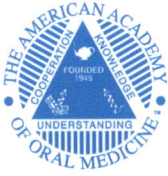

4 Intervening with Tobacco Users

HEALTH BENEFITS OF SMOKING CESSATION

Within 20 minutes of your last cigarette,
- Blood pressure drops to normal.
- Pulse rate returns to normal.
- Hand and foot temperatures increase to normal.

After 8 hours,
- Carbon monoxide level in blood returns to normal.
- The oxygen level in your blood increases to normal.

After 24 hours,
- Chance of heart attack is reduced.

After 48 hours,
- Nerve endings adjust to the absence of nicotine.
- The ability to smell and taste is enhanced.The tobacco smell on your breath is dissipated.

After 72 hours,
- Bronchial tubes relax = breathing is easier.
- Lung capacity increases.

After 2 weeks to 3 months,
- Circulation improves.
- Walking becomes easier.
- Lung function increases as much as 30%.

After 1 to 9 months,
- Smoker's cough, sinus congestion, fatigue, and shortness of breath all decrease.
- Cilia regrow in the lung, increasing the ability to handle mucus, clean the lungs, and reduce the chance of infection.
- The body's overall energy level increases.

After 1 year,
- Heart disease death rate approaches 50% of that of a nonsmoker.

After 5 years,
- Heart disease rate drops to the rate for nonsmokers.
- Lung cancer death rate decreases halfway back to that of nonsmokers.

After 10 years,
- Precancerous cells of the mouth and lungs are replaced.
- The lung cancer death rate drops to that of nonsmokers, as well as the incidence of other cancers (i.e., the mouth, larynx, esophagus, bladder, kidney,and pancreas).

ECONOMIC BENEFITS OF TOBACCO CESSATION

Aside from the health benefits associated with ceasing to smoke tobacco, there are significant monetary gains as well, as outlined in Table 4-1. The average price of a pack of cigarettes in the United States is $6.28 and by state retail price

TABLE 4 - 1: POTENTIAL SAVINGS PER YEAR OF CEASING TO SMOKE TOBACCOS ($)					
	Price Per Pack				
Packs per Day	$6.00	$7.00	$8.00	$9.00	$10.00
0.5	1,095	1,277	1,465	1,642	1,825
1	2,190	2,555	2,920	3,285	3,650
1.5	3,285	3,832	4,380	4,927	5,475
2	4,380	5,110	5,840	6,570	7,300
3	6,570	7,665	8,760	9,855	10,950

ranged from approximeately $5 in Missouri to approx. $10.5 in New York.

Intervention

Despite the sustained prevalence of tobacco use, the response of the health care professions and the health care delivery system has been disappointing. Who is to blame when providers do not receive the training or support necessary to treat tobacco use? The current treatments available to control tobacco dependence offer primary care providers a unique opportunity to reduce the loss of life and health caused by this chronic unhealthy behavior. In the past, tobacco intervention was perceived to be difficult by many health care providers. Frequently cited reasons include the following barriers:

- Lack of effective treatments
- Lack of efficacy in implementing treatments
- Inadequate time
- Inadequate reimbursement
- Poor training in tobacco cessation counseling techniques

It is the role of the dentist to inquire about tobacco use as he/she would other routine health history questions in a non-threatening, caring interpersonal atmosphere

- Be gentle when advising the patient
- Establish direct eye contact while verbalizing concerns for his/her well-being
- Personalize your advice
- Address benefits of cessation

The 2000 Public Health Service (PHS) guidelines serve as the foundation for treating tobacco dependence in the dental environment, establishing the following facts:

- Tobacco dependence is a chronic disease.
- Permanent abstinence will be achieved by a small number of patients.
  - The majority of patients will continue to use tobacco for many years, cycling through multiple periods of relapse and remission.
  - Tobacco dependence is a chronic condition that can be treated with brief interventions in the clinical dental setting.
  - Dentists should identify every tobacco user, advise users to quit, provide brief motivational counseling, and provide appropriate pharmacotherapy.

PUBLIC HEALTH SERVICE GUIDELINE

In 2000 Public Health Service (PHS) guideline listed the recommendations for effective clinical treatments for tobacco dependence as follows:

- The first step in treating tobacco use is to identify tobacco users.
  - Studies have shown that patients want and expect their health care provider to ask and advise them about their tobacco use.
  - Over 50% of adults between the ages of 18 and 55 years visit a dental office at least once per year.
  - Studies have demonstrated that showing patients oral lesions related to their tobacco use is a powerful motivator for initiating an attempt to quit.
  - Oral healthcare providers can implement interventions (Figure 4-1), as brief as 3 minutes, and be effective in increasing cessation rates.
  - Brief interventions are effective with all populations, including older smokers, pregnant women, adolescent tobacco users, and racial and ethnic minorities.

- Consideration should be given to the appropriateness of pharmacotherapy in certain populations, including
  - Patients smoking fewer than 10 cigarettes
  - Patients with certain medical conditions
  - Pregnant breast-feeding women
  - Adolescent tobacco users

- The 5 A's intervention is recommended by the National Cancer Institute and Public Health Service guidelines:
  - ASK the patient about tobacco use.
  - ADVISE the patient to quit (strong, clear message) (see Figure 4-1).
  - ASSESS the willingness of the patient to make an attempt to quit.
  - ASSIST the patient who is willing to set a "quit date" (pharmacotherapy).
  - ARRANGE for follow-up contact to prevent relapse; contact the patient 1 to 2 days prior to the quit date and 2 weeks after the quit date, and then follow up as needed.

These strategies are designed to take 3 minutes or less. A dental office that integrates the 5 A's into its existing system of care will ensure the adoption of these strategies. Every patient who wants to make an attempt to quit using tobacco should receive brief counseling, pharmacotherapy, and follow-up.

The 5 A's Brief Intervention

1. **ASK:** Systematically identify all tobacco users at every visit. Expand the database of the patient's vital signs to include the use of any form of tobacco:

Vital Signs

Blood pressure: _____ Pulse: _____

Weight: _____

Temperature: _____ Respiratory rate: _____

Tobacco use (circle one): CURRENT   FORMER   NEVER

Type of tobacco _____

Alternatives to expanding the vital signs include:

- Placing tobacco-use status stickers on all patient charts.
- Indicating tobacco-use status using electronic medical records or computer reminder systems.

2. **ADVISE:** Strongly urge all tobacco users to quit. The advice should be:

- Clear: "I think it is important for you to quit smoking now, and I can help you." "Cutting down while you are ill is not enough."
- Strong: "As your clinician, I need you to know that quitting smoking is the most important thing you can do to protect your health now and in the future. The clinic staff and I will help you."
- Personalized: Link tobacco use to current health or illness and/or its social economic costs, motivation level or readiness to quit, and/or the impact of tobacco use on children and others in the household.

3. **ASSESS:** Determine the willingness to make an attempt to quit:

- If the patient is willing to make an attempt to quit at this time, provide assistance.
- If the patient will participate in an intensive treatment, deliver such a treatment or refer to an intensive intervention.
- If patient is unwilling to make a quit attempt, provide motivational intervention (see 5 R's).

4. **ASSIST:** Aid the patient in quitting:

- Set a quit date; ideally, the quit date should be within 2 weeks.

- Encourage the patient to:
  - Tell family, friends, and coworkers about quitting and request understanding and support.
  - Anticipate challenges (nicotine withdrawal) to a planned quit attempt, particularly during the critical first few weeks.
  - Remove tobacco products from your environment. Prior to quitting, avoid smoking in places where you spend a lot of time (eg, work, home, car).
  - Avoid situational cues, such as alcohol consumption or socializing with active smokers, which may facilitate unplanned relapse.
  - Provide motivational literature.
  - Consider pharmacotherapy.

Pharmacotherapy General Overview

- U.S. Food and Drug Administration (FDA)-approved pharmaceuticals are safe and effective when used as directed.
- The choice of medication varies with each patient, as does the tailoring of motivational support and building of coping skills.
- Current recommendations call for 2 to 3 months of pharmacotherapy. During this time, patients can and should learn to cope with high-risk situations without having to experience severe nicotine withdrawal.
- FDA-approved pharmaceuticals, used in combination with a behavioral intervention, increase long-term (6 months or longer) abstinence rates compared with a behavioral intervention alone.
- All FDA-approved pharmaceuticals are for adult smokers. (Expert opinion is that comparable use is probably appropriate for smokeless tobacco users.)
- In general, nicotine replacement therapy should be discontinued for individuals who continue to use tobacco.
- The provider must be vigilant for any pharmacologic interactions between nicotine replacement therapy use and other medications. Certain drugs have an increased effect when nicotine is present, whereas others have a decreased effect.When the patient stops all nicotine, other medication dosages should be accordingly adjusted.

Numerous pharmacotherapies for smoking cessation now exist. Except in the presence of contraindications, these should be used with patients attempting to quit smoking.

Key Guideline Recommendations

Tobacco dependence is a chronic condition that often requires repeated intervention. However, effective treatments exist that can produce long-term or even permanent abstinence:

- Because effective tobacco dependence treatments are available, every patient who uses tobacco should be offered at least one of these treatments:
  - Patients willing to try to quit tobacco use should be provided with treatments identified as effective in this guideline.
  - Patients unwilling to try to quit tobacco use should be provided with a brief intervention designed to increase their motivation to quit.
- It is essential that clinicians and health care delivery systems (including administrators, insurers, and purchasers) institutionalize the consistent identification, documentation, and treatment of every tobacco user seen in their health care setting.
- Brief tobacco dependence treatment is effective, and every patient who uses tobacco should be offered at least brief treatment.
- There is a strong dose-response relationship between the intensity of tobacco dependence counseling and its effectiveness. Treatments involving person-to-person contact (via individual, group, or proactive telephone counseling) are consistently effective, and their effectiveness increases with treatment intensity (eg, minutes of contact).
- Three types of counseling and behavioral therapies were found to be especially effective and should be used with all patients attempting tobacco cessation:
  - Provision of practical counseling (problem solving/skills training)
  - Provision of social support as part of treatment (intratreatment social support)
  - Help in securing social support outside treatment (extratreatment social support)
- Numerous effective pharmacotherapies for smoking cessation now exist. Except in the presence of contraindications, these should be used with patients attempting to quit smoking:
  - Six first-line pharmacotherapies are identified that reliably increase long-term smoking abstinence rates:
    - Nicotine transdermal (patch)
    - Nicotine polacrilex (gum)
    - Nicotine inhaler
    - Nicotine nasal spray
    - Nicotine lozenge
    - Bupropion SR
- Two second-line pharmacotherapies are identified as efficacious and may be considered by clinicians if first-line pharmacotherapies are not effective:
  - Nortriptyline
  - Clonidine
- Over-the-counter nicotine patches are effective relative to placebo, and their use should be encouraged.
- Contraindications for nicotine replacement products include:
  - Under age 18
  - Women who are pregnant or nursing (nicotine gum is FDA approved for use in pregnancy)
  - Immediate post-myocardial infarction period
  - Severe arrythmia
  - severe or worsening angina pectoris
- Tobacco dependence treatments are both clinically effective and costeffective relative to other medical and disease prevention interventions. As such, insurers and purchasers should ensure that:
  - All insurance plans include as a reimbursed benefit the counseling and pharmacotherapeutic treatments identified as effective in this guideline.
  - Clinicians are reimbursed for providing tobacco dependence treatment, just as they are reimbursed for treating other chronic conditions.

5. **ARRANGE:** Schedule follow-up contact:
- Timing: Follow-up contact should occur soon after the quit date, preferably during the first week. A second follow-up contact is recommended within the first month. Schedule further follow-up contacts as indicated. A postcard or telephone call is appropriate.

- Actions during follow-up contact: Congratulate success. If tobacco use has occurred, review the circumstances and encourage recommitment to total abstinence. Remind the patient that a lapse can be used as a learning experience. Identify problems already encountered and anticipate challenges in the immediate future. Assess pharmacotherapy use and problems. Consider use or referral to more intensive treatment.

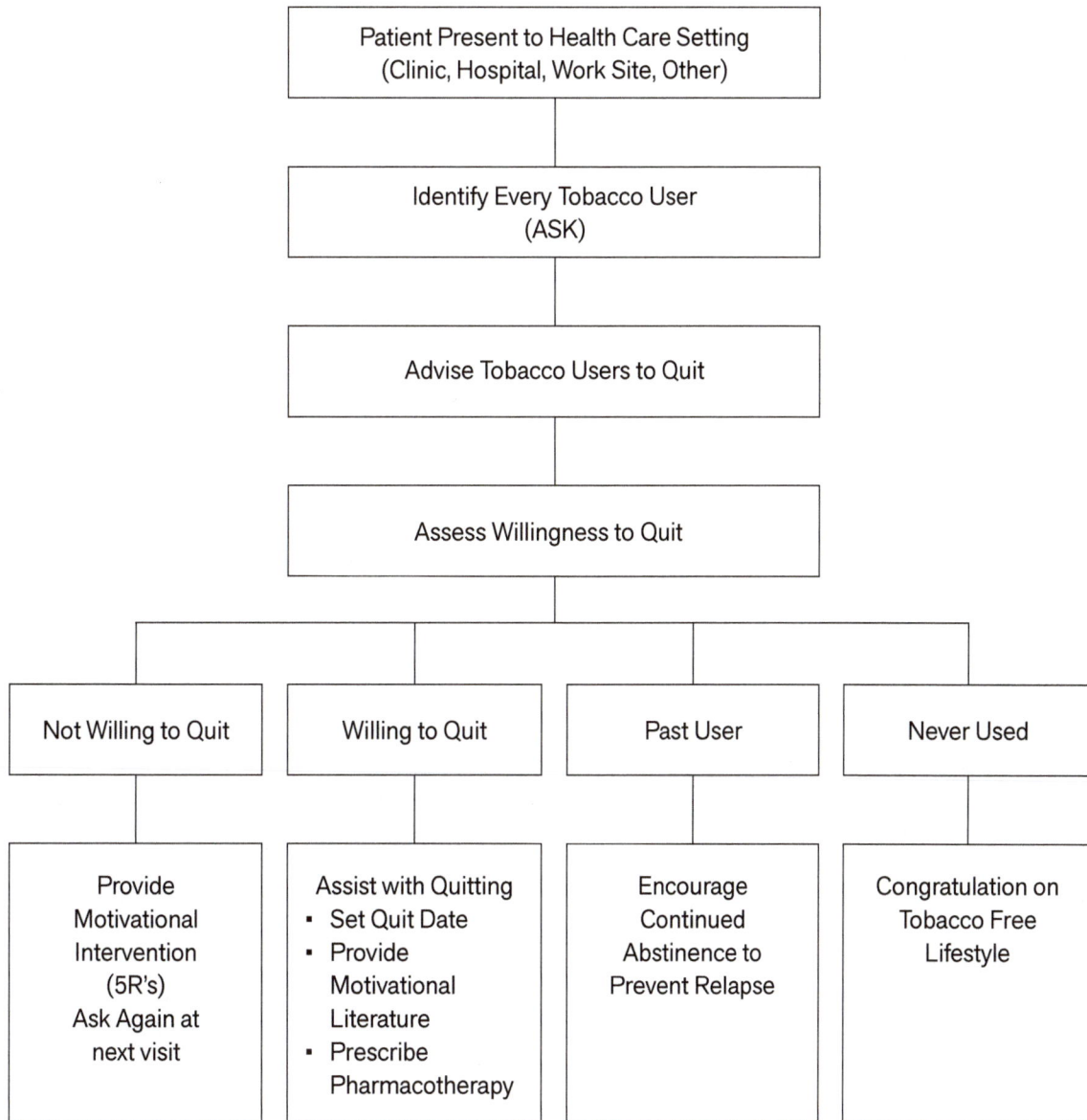

Figure 4–1: *Intervention algorithm for treating tobacco use. Relapse prevention interventions are not necessary in the case of the adult who has not used tobacco for many years*

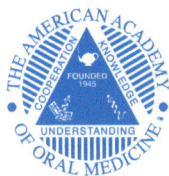

5 Pharmacotherapy for Tobacco Cessation: Specific Medications

Expressing interest in smoking cessation by the patient is the first step in smoking cessation.The highest success rates for smoking cessation in a motivated patient are achieved by a combination of pharmacologic therapies, cognitive and behavioral therapies. With regards to pharmacologic therapies nicotine replacement therapy, bupropion (antidepressant) and varenicline (partial nicotine agonist) are FDA approved for smoking cessation. Other medications used off-label for smoking cessation include nortriptyline, cytisine and clonidine.

NICOTINE REPLACEMENT THERAPY (NRT)

Indications

Nicotine replacement products were developed to reduce or eliminate withdrawal symptoms. They provide assistance for individuals interested in quitting to plan for and deal with the psychological and behavioral (social) components of their nicotine addiction. Prescribing combination nicotine replacement products results in higher smoking cessation rates than single-product therapies. Nicotine replacement products should be prescribed in conjunction with the patient's general practitioner.

Contraindications

Should severe or worsening of angina pectoris develop, these products should be discontinued. Use caution with patients who have hyperthyroidism, insulin-dependent diabetes and active peptic ulcers. Stable coronary artery disease is not a contraindication.

Nicotine Transdermal Patch

Nicotine patches may help patients stop by allowing them to cope with the social and psychological aspects of not using tobacco without experiencing nicotine withdrawal. Nicotine patches provide continuous, long-acting, slow release nicotine delivery. Although compliance with nicotine patches is high, patients seldom are successful in stopping tobacco use when using nicotine patches in the absence of appropriate counseling and follow-up. Dentists should have

tobacco cessation brochures and treatment plans in their offices that include such counseling services. Transdermal nicotine is well tolerated systemically and topically. The most commonly reported side effects are temporary itching, burning, and/or erythema at the application site. The dose-related adverse effects of transdermal nicotine therapy are mild to moderate sleep disturbance (e.g., insomnia and abnormal, vivid dreams), dyspepsia, various myalgias, body aches, and cough. The incidence of almost all side effects decreases after a few days of treatment. Fewer than 5% of tobacco users discontinue patch use as a result of side effects. Nicotine patches are available over-the-counter in the US.

Instructions

Tobacco cessation must be initiated prior to using nicotine patches. This patch is applied once every 24 hours to a nonhairy, clean, dry site on the upper body or arm. The skin site should not be reused for at least 1 week. Different brands vary in nicotine dose and recommended length of use. All brands recommend a higher dose (21–22 mg) for the first 6 weeks and then use lower-dose patches 14mg/day for 2 weeks followed by 7mg/day for another 2 weeks A lower initial dose may be used for patients with cardiovascular disease or those weighing less than 100 pounds.

> **Rx**: Nicotine transdermal patch (21–22 mg).
> Disp: One patch daily for 6 weeks (42 patches).
> Sig: Tobacco cessation must be initiated prior to using nictone patches. Apply once every 24 hours to a nonhairy, clean, dry site on the upper body or arm. Skin site should not be reused for at least 1 week

Contraindications

People under the age of 18 years should not use the patch, nor should women who are pregnant or nursing or patients who are immediate post–myocardial infarction. Patients with severe arrhythmia or uncontrolled or worsening angina pectoris should not use this product. Caution is advised with hyperthyroidism, pheochromocytoma, insulin-dependent diabetes, active peptic ulcers, uncontrolled severe blood pressure, severe skin conditions, and kidney or liver disease.

Nicotine Gum

Nicotine gum is a very commonly used short-acting nicotine replacement product that is used in combination with nicotine patches to control withdrawl symptoms. The nicotine that is released following chewing is readily absorbed via the oral mucosa producing a systemic effect with peak nicotine blood levels occurring approximately after 20 minutes. It is recommended that heavy smokers (>25 cigarettes daily) use the 4 mg dose and the 2 mg dose is advised for lighter smokers. The patient is advised to chew the nicotine gum whenever there is an urge to smoke. Reduced nicotine absorption may occur if the oral pH is lowered from coffee, carbonated drinks or acidic beverages. Therefore the use of these beverages, before or during nicotine gum use, is best avoided.

> **Rx**: Nicorette (Nicotine gum), 2-4 mg.
> Disp: 200 pieces of 2 or 4 mg daily for 6 months, then gradually reduce.
> Sig: No smoking or smokeless tobacco while using nicotine gum. No acidic or hot beverages during or immediately before using Nicorette (eg, soft drinks, fruit juices, milk, beer, coffee, or tea). Nicorette is not chewed like regular gum. Chew very slowly until you sense a peppery taste or feel a slight tingling in your mouth; then stop chewing and "park" the Nicorette between cheek and gums. After the taste or tingling is almost gone (about 1 minute), chew slowly again until the taste or tingling returns; then stop chewing and park the Nicorette again using a different location in the mouth. Chew each piece for 20 to 30 minutes and discard. Use adequate amounts, depending on addiction stage.

Contraindications

People under 18 years should not use nicotine gum. Those in the immediate post–myocardial infarction, individuals with life-threatening arrhythmia, and people with severe or worsening angina should abstain. Also, people with active temporomandibular disorders should not use this product. Those who are pregnant or considering pregnancy should not use nicotine gum. Use with caution in patients with hyperthyroidism or insulin-dependent diabetes.

Side Effects

Gastrointestinal distress, hiccups, nausea, gas (from chewing too fast), jaw ache, cheek biting, oral irritation, and sialorrhea may result from nicotine gum use.

Nicotine Lozenges

Nicotine lozenges are another commonly used short-acting nicotine replacement product that may be used in combination with nicotine patches to control withdrawal symptoms. Nicotine lozenges are easier to use than nicotine gum and may be preferable in patients who suffer from temporomandibular dysfunction. The patient is instructed to allow the lozenge to dissolve in the mouth for 30 minutes. The higher dose of 4 mg is recommended for smokers with a greater nicotine dependence.

Side Effects

Gastrointestinaldistress,nausea,vomiting, diarrhea, headache, heart palpitations, and oral irritation.

> **Rx**: *Commit* (nicotine lozenge), 2 or 4 mg.
> Disp: 72 lozenges, 2 or 4 mg.
> Sig: Use when the urge to smoke creates uncontrolled cravings. Place one lozenge in the mouth and let it slowly dissolve, occasionally changing its position. Do not smoke or use smokeless tobacco while using Commit. Do not use more than one lozenge at a time or continuously use one lozenge after the other. Do not eat or drink 15 minutes before using or while the stop-smoking lozenge is in your mouth. Do not use more than five lozenges in 6 hours or more than 20 lozenges total per day.

Nicotine Inhaler

Nicotine inhalers are capable of producing plasma nicotine levels equal to one third of that of conventional cigarettes. Six to 16 nicotine-containing cartridges daily is the recommended dose for the first three months and then this dose may be reduced as tolerated.

Side Effects

Throat irritation and bronchospasm may occur.

Nicotine nasal spray

Nicotine nasal sprays produce higher levels of plasma nicotine than other nicotine replacement products with peak nicotine levels being achieved after 10 minutes of use. 1-2 sprays per hour is the recommended dose for the first three months. The recommended maximum daily dose is 80 sprays.

Side Effects

Nasal and throat irritation, epiphora and rhinitis may occur.

Other Nicotine Replacement Products

Nicotine mouth sprays and nicotine sublingual tablets are other short-acting nicotine replacement products however these products are not available in the US.

Electronic Cigarettes (E-Cigarettes)

E-cigarettes are battery-powered electronic delivery systems that heat a liquid containing nicotine, aerosolizing nicotine into a vapor that is then inhaled. E-cigarettes first entered the US markets in 2006 and were not tightly regulated. It is unclear at this time how e-cigarettes will influence national smoking prevalence rates and whether e-cigarettes may potentially be used by children as a gateway to conventional cigarettes. Their use as a smoking cessation aid at this juncture is controversial and clinical trials are currently ongoing. In 2016 the FDA had not approved e-cigarettes as a smoking cessation aid due to safety and efficacy concerns. Although, e-cigarettes are likely less harmful than conventional cigarettes, recent studies demonstrate that e-cigarettes still contain carcinogens and therefore, advocating their use as a smoking cessation tool in the presence of various other available carcinogen-free FDA-approved smoking cessation aids is medicolegally ill-advised.

ANTIDEPRESSANTS

These paharamcologic agents may br in patients that have failed with NRT and provides an alternative to nicotine based treatments. When NRT was compared to bupropion results showed equal efficacy.

BUPROPION (*Zyban*)

Zyban is chemically unrelated to tricyclic, tetracyclic, or selective serotinin reuptake inhibitors or any other known antidepressant agents. *Zyban* is a non-nicotine aid to help people who want to quit smoking. It was initially developed and marketed as an antidepressant (*Wellbutrin*

Rx: *Zyban* (150 mg tablet).
Disp: 182 tablets.
Sig: Start taking *Zyban* 1 week before you stop smoking. Take one tablet in the morning for 3 days and then take two tablets per day (one in the morning and one at least 8 hours later) for up to 3 months. It may be taken with or without food. Never take an extra dose of *Zyban*.

[bupropion hydrochloride]). It is presumed to act on the dopaminergic and/or noradrenergic pathways involved in nicotine addiction and withdrawal.

Contraindications

If patients have had seizures, epilepsy or a family history of epilepsy, significant head trauma, stroke, brain tumor, or surgery then they should not use *Zyban*. Other contraindications are eating disorders (bulimia or anorexia) and taking *Wellbutrin* or *Wellbutrin* SR antidepressants or monoamine oxidase inhibitor antidepressants. *Zyban* should not be taken with other agents that may lower seizure threshold (e.g., antipsychotics, other antidepressants, theophylline, and systemic steroids) or with Parkinson's disease medication.

Side Effects

Some side effects are difficulty in sleeping, dry mouth, headache, drowsiness, decreased appetite, dizziness, sweating, nausea, an increased or irregular heart beat, and agitation or anxiety.

Dose Instructions

Start taking *Zyban* a week before you stop smoking. The initial dose is one 150 mg tablet in the morning for 3 days. Then take two tablets per day, one 150 mg tab in the morning and one 150 mg tab at least 8 hours later. The length of treatment will vary from 7 to 12 weeks. It may be taken with or without food. NEVER take an "extra" dose of *Zyban*.

NORTRIPTYLINE

Nortriptyline is a tricyclic antidepressant used off-label for smoking cessation and is considered as a second line treatment option.

Rx: Nortriptyline (25 mg tablet).
Disp: 380 tablets.
Sig: Start taking 25 mg once daily intiated 10-28 days prior to quite date and titrate to 75-100 mg/day. Continue therapy for at least 12 weeks after quit day.

Contraindications

Patients who have hypersensitivity to nortriptyline and to medications with a similar chemical class (or any component of the formulation). Patients with a history of a recent MI and are in the acute recovery phase. Patients taking monoamine oxidase inhibitor antidepressants and is not to be prescribed concurrently or within 14 days of discontinuing either one of the medications. Other contraindications include patients receiving linezolid or intravenous methylene blue.

Side Effects
Some side effects are difficulty in sleeping, dry mouth, nausea, vomiting, decreased appetite, constipation, and agitation or anxiety.

Dose Instructions
Start taking nortriptyline 10-28 days before you stop smoking ("quit day"). The initial dose is one 25 mg tablet. Increase the dose gradually until reaching a therapeutic dose of 75-100 mg. The length of treatment will be at least 12 weeks after "quit day."

GERIATRIC PATIENTS
Older people are more sensitive to anticholinergic, sedative, cardiovascular medications, as well as side effects of antidepressants as a result of renal and hepatic problems. There is no evidence that age in itself is a consideration in establishing dosing strengths and schedules (see Table 5-1).

PARTIAL NICOTINE AGONIST
Varenicline (*Chantix*)

Varenicline is a selective nicotine receptor partial agonist FDA approved as a first line treatment option for smoking cessation. Varenicline was found to be more effective than single NRT and bupropion but not more effective than combination NRT.

> **Rx**: Nortriptyline (0.5 mg tablet).
> Disp: 55 tablets.
> Sig: Start taking 0.5 mg once daily for 3 days. Then take 0.5 mg twice daily from days 4 -7. Thereafter a maintenance dose of 1 mg twice daily for 11 weeks.

Contraindications
Hypersensitivity reactions or skin reaction to any component of the formulation

Side Effects
May cause CNS depression and impair mental and physical abilities and must be cautioned. Depression and suicidal thoughts have been reported. Other side effects include nausea, and hypersensitivity reactions including erythema multiforme and Steven-Johnson syndrome

Dose Instructions
Start taking varenicline 0.5 mg once daily for days 1-3. Then take 0.5 mg twice daily for days 4 -7. A maintenance dose of 1 mg twice daily is to be maintained for 11 weeks. If dose is not tolerated a reduction may be considered.

TABLE 5 - 1: PHARMACOTHERAPY FOR TOBACCO USE: SPECIFIC MEDICATIONS			
Medication	*Proper Use*	*Advantages*	*Disadvantages*
First-line options			
Nicotine Transdermal Patch (*Nicoderm, Nicotrol, Habitrol*)	Stop tobacco 1 per day, on awakening 9 – 12 weeks Tapering option	Effective blood levels within 1–2 hours Simple to use; 3 dose levels No new drug; Eliminates "tar" and CO Concern re: use with tobacco overstated	Skin-related side effects common Caution with CV disease Max dose may not be enough for some
Nicotine Polacrilex ("gum") (*Nicorette*)	Stop tobacco Chew minimally and park for 30 minutes 1 piece every 1–2 hours Up to 24 pieces per day 12 weeks	2 mg (up to 24 cigs per day) 4mg (25 or more cigs per day) Oral/Mint/Regular Oral substitute; Use as needed Good for 'irregular' smoker	Insufficeint use is common Chewing too much increases side effects Taste can be unpleasant (original flavor) No food or drink before or while using.

TABLE 5 - 1: PHARMACOTHERAPY FOR TOBACCO USE: SPECIFIC MEDICATIONS			
Medication	**Proper Use**	**Advantages**	**Disadvantages**
Nicotine inhaler (*Nicotrol*)	Stop tobacco 6 – 16 cartridges per day 12 weeks; can taper over 6 – 12 additional weeks Stop if not quit in 4 weeks	Easy to tailor Oral substitute	Lower level of delivery — may not be ideal for heavier users as sole therapy Costly
Nicotine Nasal Spray (*Nicotrol NS*)	Stop tobacco 1 – 2 doses per hour (I dose = 1 spray in each nostril) Max: 5 doses per hour (40 doeses per day) Do not inhale while spraying 12 weeks Stop if not quit in 4 weeks	May be more useful in heavier users	Irritation of nasal tract Costly
Nicotine Lozenge (*Commit*)	Stop tobacco Absorbed via oral mucosa Not eating or drinking 15 minutes before use Up to 6 per 5-hour period, max of 20 per day 12 weeks	2 mg (1st cigarette after 30 min of awakening) 4 mg (1st cigarette sooner than 30 min) Oral substitute Use as needed Good for "irregular" smokers	Consuming too fast can cause side effects No food or drink before or while using
Bupropion SR (*Zyban*)	Once per day for 3days, then twice per day for at least 7 – 12 weeks (up to 6 months) Tapering at end of treatment not necessary	Ease of use Can initiate while still using tobacco Antidepressant effect	h/o seizures or eating disorder Abrupt stopping of alcohol, sedatives No MAOI or other form of Bupropion 1 – 2 weeks to reach adequate blood levels
Varenicline (FDA-approved) (*Chantix*) Second-line options	Monitor closely 0.5 mg daily for 3 days followed by 0.5 mg daily for 4 days followed by 1 mg BID for 12 weeks	Highest abstinence rates compared to all other agents	FDA *black box warning* for potential neuropsychiatric side effects. Significant risk for cardiovascular patients
Notriptyline (not FDA-approved)	Monitor closely 25 mg/day; gradual increase to 75-100 mg/day for 12 weeks	3x increase in abstinence over placebo	Higher level of side effects. Significant risk for cardiovascular patients
Clonidine (not FDA-approved)	Monitor closely PO: 0.10 mg/day; increase by 0.10 mg/day as needed up to 0.75 mg/day TTS: 0.10 mg/day; increase to 0.20 mg/day as needed 3-10 weeks	2x abstinence rates compared with placebo Transdermal or oral	Higher level of side effects, especially with abrupt discontinuation
FDA = US Food and Drug Administration; MAOI = monoamine oxidase inhibitor; PO = orally.			

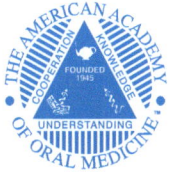

6 Patients Who Are Not Ready to Make a Quit Attempt

Dentists should provide a brief intervention to help motivate the patient to quit. Patients may lack the information about the harmful effects of tobacco on their oral and systemic health. They also may have fears or concerns about quitting because of past failure attempts. Many tobacco using patients lack the financial resources.

These patients may respond in a positive way to a motivational message that reassures and educates them. Dentists can enhance their motivational intervention by engaging in a supportive, empathetic relationship with their patient that focuses on the patient's efforts rather than the outcomes. Because of the chronic relapsing nature of tobacco dependence, recent quitters need continual positive reinforcement. Although most relapses occur early in the quitting process, it can occur months and possibly years after the quit date

COMPONENTS OF THE 5 R'S IN TOBACCO CESSATION
- Relevance
- Risk
- Rewards
- Roadblocks
- Reputation

Relevance
Encourage the patient to indicate why quitting is personally relevant, being as specific as possible. Motivational information has the greatest impact if it is relevant to a patient's disease status or risk, family or social situation (e.g., having children in the home), health concerns, age, sex, and other important patient characteristics (e.g., previous quitting experience, personal barriers to cessation).

Risks
The clinician should ask the patient to identify the potential negative consequences of tobacco use. The clinician may suggest and highlight those that seem most relevant to the patient. The clinician should emphasize that smoking low tar and/or low-nicotine cigarettes or use of other forms of tobacco (eg, smokeless tobacco, cigars, and pipes) will not eliminate these risks. The following are examples of risks:

- Acute risks: shortness of breath, exacerbation of asthma, harm to pregnancy, impotence, infertility, increased serum carbon monoxide levels
- Long-term risks: myocardial infarction, strokes, lung and other cancers (larynx, oral cavity, pharynx, esophagus, pancreas, bladder, cervix), chronic obstructive pulmonary diseases (chronic bronchitis and emphysema), longterm disability, and need for extended care
- Environmental risks: increased risk of lung cancer and heart disease in spouses; higher rates of smoking by children of tobacco users; increased risk of low birth weight, sudden infant death syndrome, asthma, middle ear disease, and respiratory infections in children of smokers; harmful effects to pets

REWARDS
The clinician should ask the patient to identify the potential benefits of stopping tobacco use. The clinician may suggest and highlight those that seem most relevant to the patient. Examples of rewards include improved health; food will taste better; improved sense of smell; saving money; feeling better about yourself; home, car, clothing, and breath will appear cleaner and smell better; can stop worrying about quitting; setting a good example for children; having healthier babies and children; not worrying about exposing others to smoke; feeling better physically; performing better in physical activities; reduced wrinkling and aging of skin. The definitive economic benefits of tobacco cessation should be emphasized. (see Table 4-1)

Roadblocks
The clinician should ask the patient to identify barriers or impediments to quitting and note elements of treatment (problem solving, pharmacotherapy) that could address

barriers. Typical barriers might include withdrawal symptoms, fear of failure, weight gain, lack of support, depression, and enjoyment of tobacco.

Repetition

The motivational intervention should be repeated every time an unmotivated patient visits the clinical setting. Tobacco users who have failed in previous quit attempts should be told that most people make repeated attempts to quit before they are successful.

Tobacco dependence has many features of a chronic disease and that failure to recognize this may undermine a clinician's motivation to treat tobacco use. Epidemiologic data have shown that more than 70% of the 50 million smokers in America have made at least one previous attempt to quit and approximately 45% will try to quit each year. Most of these attempts will be unsuccessful. By identifying every smoker, advising smokers to quit, assessing readiness to make an attempt, assisting with the attempt to quit (setting a quit date, motivational literature, pharmacotherapy), and arranging for follow-up, the oral health care team will achieve 12 to 15% 1-year abstinence rates that, compared with the self-quit rate of 2 to 4%, are substantial.

SUGGESTIONS FOR QUITTING TOBACCO USE

Nicotine, the active agent in all tobacco products, is a highly addictive drug. The objective of the use of any form of tobacco is the delivery of a small dose of nicotine to the brain, producing a desirable effect. When an individual takes a puff on a cigarette, his or her brain quickly gets the message that it wants more of the chemicals that it is being given. That is why quitting smoking is just as hard, sometimes harder, than getting off drugs such as alcohol, cocaine, or heroin. For the long-term tobacco user, quitting can be a real challenge because it involves both behavior (habit) and addiction (biochemical dependence). Fortunately, tobacco users can be assisted with behavior modification and with several medications.

For nicotine replacement therapy, nicotine gum, skin patches, nasal sprays, lozenges and inhalers are among the agents that have worked well for many exsmokers. The non-nicotine pill Zyban (bupropion hydrochloride) can reduce the urge to smoke and may make quitting easier.

Some of these products are available over the counter at retail drugstores. Healthcare providers and other former smokers can be of great help when you are preparing to quit. They often know what to expect, how to plan, and what works and what does not work in various situations.

TAKING THE FIRST STEPS AFTER YOU HAVE DECIDED TO QUIT

Plan how you will quit. Ask your doctor for help.

- Set a quit date.

- Tell your family, friends, and coworkers that you are going to quit and when.

- Ask them for support and understanding. Smoking spouses should mutually agree to quit.

- Change your environment. That means getting rid of cigarettes and ashtrays in your home, car, and workplace. Avoid all social, recreational, and occupational situations where you might be exposed to the sight and smell of tobacco products.

- Change your habits. Try not to smoke in places where you spend a lot of time, such as your home or car.

- Review previous attempts and failures to quit. Think about what worked and what did not work for you. Be prepared to manage stressful situations without the use of tobacco.

- When your quit date arrives, stop smoking completely, beginning as you awake in the morning. The first few days are usually the hardest, so concentrate on stopping for just 1 day at a time. Congratulate and reward yourself often for your successes.

- Remind yourself that quitting is hard. Although most people need two or more attempts before they finally succeed, studies have shown that each time you try, you become stronger and learn more about what helps and what does not help. If you start smoking again, rethink your plan and start fresh. Right now, half of all people who ever smoked have quit. You can too!

Stop-smoking medications can help.

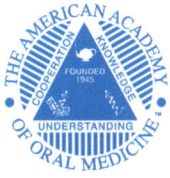

7 What to Say to Your Tobacco-Using Patient

USE AND CESSATION

The stage has been set for dental professionals to become actively involved as facilitators and leaders in tobacco education efforts. Currently, an increasing number of dentists, hygienists, and assistants are participating in clinical and community interventions that focus on both prevention and cessation strategies. The public has also become accustomed to receiving "sound bites"—straightforward messages about health issues, delivered in ways that are simple to recall and reflect on.

As an Oral Health Professional, What Do I Say to Patients about Smoking and Tobacco Cessation?

Many practitioners want to know what messages will have the most impact and how they can be delivered in a meaningful and effective way. An effective cessation message focuses on the benefits of becoming a nonsmoker rather than the detriments of continuing to smoke. However, when responding to this perspective, some smokers may rationalize that the damage caused by their smoking is already done. In keeping with a positive theme of hope, the practitioner can say,

- "It is never too late to quit smoking."

- "When you quit, most of the effects of smoking are reversible."

- "Smoking cessation is the single most important step that you can take to enhance the length and quality of your life."

- "Your mouth will be a lot healthier and fresher when you quit smoking."

- "When you quit smoking, you will no longer be inhaling more than 4,000 harmful chemicals and gases."

Make Your Message Relevant

It is critically important for dentists and hygienists to interact with patients who smoke and to carefully explain how their specific dental problems are linked to their smoking behaviors. For example, during treatment, if the dental hygienist notes an oral condition related to tobacco use, not only can the hygienist discuss the problem with the patient, he or she can also encourage the patient to observe this condition by using a hand mirror. Additionally, the dental hygienist can assess the individual's readiness to set a quit date. Through discussion with the hygienist and a review of well-documented notes (kept in the treatment record), the dentist can make a diagnosis and arrange for appropriate follow-up. As they gain experience in discussing tobacco issues with patients, oral health professionals can become as comfortable with cessation issues as they are with details concerning periodontal pocket depths and plaque control.

During subsequent appointments, as dental health care providers interact with their patients who smoke, they can relay the following messages:

- "As your dentist (hygienist), I must advise you to stop smoking now."

- "Have you ever thought about quitting? Have you ever tried to stop before?" If so, "What happened?"

- "Did you know that you have periodontal disease? Quitting smoking would really help slow down the rate of gum disease that is developing in your mouth."

- "You need to have gum surgery, but you will not heal properly unless you quit smoking."

- "Smoking is a common cause of bad breath. You may be able to solve this problem completely if you quit using cigarettes."

- "How about choosing a quit date within the next few weeks, now that you have decided to stop smoking?"

Fear of Weight Gain

The fear of weight gain discourages many smokers (especially women) from trying to quit. Weight issues should be acknowledged and dealt with openly. The following responses may help diffuse weight issues:

- "Did you know that as many as a third of people who quit smoking do not gain any weight? And those who do generally gain only 5 to 9 pounds."

- "The health risks that you are taking by smoking are far greater than the risk of nominal weight gain."

- "If you exercise regularly, you can ease withdrawal symptoms and counteract weight gain."

- "Now that you have given up smoking and want to eat more often, you need to avoid high-calorie snacks. Many of the foods that are good for oral health will also help you avoid weight gain. Be careful about substituting high-sugar items such as gum or breath mints for tobacco."

Encourage individuals with weight gain concerns to closely monitor their calorie, sugar, and fat intake and to increase their activity levels. Regular exercise not only speeds metabolism, tones muscles, improves cardiovascular functions, reduces tension, and burns calories. It also stimulates the release of endorphins, which can positively affect mood and disposition.

Although general health gains resulting from smoking cessation are well documented and dramatic, the psychological benefits associated with quitting are equally valid and impressive. Compared with current smokers, former smokers have a greater sense of self-efficacy, freedom, and control over their personal circumstances.

The following supportive comments may motivate the patient who smokes to make a commitment to cessation:

- "It sounds to me as if you would like to regain control of your life again by quitting smoking. That's a worthy goal!"

- "Just think of all the freedom you'll have when you quit! Every cigarette that you do not smoke represents a bit of freedom that you have gained."

Encouragement can be offered to patients from a health professional who is a former smoker:

- "Although this has been one of the most difficult tasks that I have ever accomplished as an adult, it is one of the most satisfying things I have ever done."

- "More than 3 million Americans quit every year. In fact, there are now 46 million of us who are ex-smokers. I can

tell you from personal experience that it can be done. Why not give it a try? I will be here to support you."

This emphatic response can be given to smokers who tried to quit but did not achieve cessation:

- "I really respect the fact that you gave quitting a good try. Not everyone succeeds on their first try, but many people are able to quit after making several attempts. Why not try again?"

Cost of Smoking

Although very few people quit smoking to save money, they are quite surprised to discover the actual cost of their tobacco use. (see Table 4-1) The following comments are examples of how a health professional might motivate a resistant smoker to a state of cessation readiness:

- "Do you realize that, as a pack-a-day smoker, you are spending over $700 a year on your addiction?"

- "When you smoke, you pay three times: first, with your money; second, with your health; and third, with more money as you try to regain your health."

- "When you quit smoking, why not set aside the money that you would have spent on cigarettes and on your first anniversary as a nonsmoker reward yourself with a special gift?"

Smokers' Rights

In reaction to any form of cessation advice, some smokers will say, "It's my right to smoke if I want to!" (This notion of smoking as an expression of personal choice and freedom is openly encouraged by the tobacco industry.) The health professional needs to diffuse this attitude by responding with acceptance and empathy:

- "Of course, it's your right. A lot of people share your view. As a health care provider, I have been taught to look at smoking as a health issue. Tell me more about your viewpoint."

- "I believe that people need to have their own reasons for wanting to quit. You have to act on your own desire to quit and not on the wishes of somebody else."

- "If you're not ready to quit just now, I understand. The choice is yours. If you ever decide that you do want to give it a try, let me know. I'll be willing to help you."

Although dental professionals need to accept each smoker's present state of readiness, they can also discretely suggest a cessation plan, even before a quit decision has been made. By taking this stance, these facilitators are fulfilling their ethical obligation without pressuring for an immediate response. The seed has now been planted. Eventually, some smokers will seek cessation help, especially when they know that a caring, nonjudgmental health professional is willing to guide them toward recovery.

QUESTIONS FREQUENTLY ASKED BY TOBACCO USERS AND THEIR ANSWERS

Q: Why should I quit?
A: You will live longer and feel better. Quitting will lower your chances of having a heart attack, stroke, or cancer. The people you live with, especially children, will be healthier. If you are pregnant, you will improve your chances of having a healthy baby. And you will have extra money to spend on things other than cigarettes.

Q: What is the first thing I need to do once I've decided to quit?
A: You should set a quit date—the day when you will break free of your tobacco addiction. Then consider visiting your dentist or other health care provider before the quit date. He or she can help by providing practical advice and information on the medication that is best for you.

Q: What medication would work best for me?
A: Different people do better with different methods. You have five choices of medications that are currently approved by the US Food and Drug Administration: a nonnicotine pill (*Wellbutrin SR* [bupropion]), nicotine gum, a nicotine inhaler, a nicotine nasal spray, nicotine lozenge and a nicotine patch. The gum and patches are available at your local pharmacy, or you can ask your health care provider to write you a prescription for one of the other medications. The good news is that all six medications have been shown to be effective in helping smokers who are motivated to quit.

Q: How will I feel when I quit smoking? Will I gain weight?
A: Many smokers gain weight when they quit, but it is usually less than 10 pounds. Eat a healthy diet, stay active, and try not to let weight gain distract you from your main goal—quitting smoking. Some of the medications to help you quit may help delay weight gain.

Q: Some of my friends and family are smokers. What should I do when I'm with them?
A: Tell them that you are quitting and ask them to assist you in this effort. Specifically, ask them not to smoke or leave cigarettes around you.

Q: What kinds of activities can I do when I feel the urge to smoke?
A: Talk with someone, go for a walk, drink water, or get busy with a task. Reduce your stress by taking a hot bath, exercising, or reading a book.

Q: How can I change my daily routine, which includes smoking a cigarette with my breakfast?
A: When you first try to quit, change your routine. Eat breakfast in a different place and drink tea instead of coffee. Take a different route to work.

Q: I like to smoke when I have a drink. Do I have to give up both?
A: It's best to avoid drinking alcohol for the first 3 months after quitting because drinking lowers your chances of success at quitting. It helps to drink a lot of water and other nonalcoholic drinks when you are trying to quit.

Q: I've tried to quit before and it didn't work. What can I do?
A: Remember that most people try to quit at least 2 or 3 times before they are successful. Review your past attempts to quit. Think about what worked—and what didn't—and try to use your most successful strategies again.

Q: What should I do if I need more help?
A: Get individual, group, or telephone counseling. The more counseling you get, the better your chances are of quitting for good. Programs are given at local hospitals and health centers. Call your local health department for information about programs in your area. Also, talk with your doctor or other health care provider.

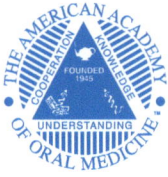

8 Using Dental Codes for Tobacco Counseling for the Control and Prevention of Tobacco-Related Disease

DENTAL CODE [CD-2] #01320: TOBACCO COUNSELING FOR THE CONTROL AND PREVENTION OF ORAL DISEASE

Dental Office–Based Tobacco Cessation Concepts that Apply to All Tobacco Patients

The oral health team should heighten cessation awareness and motivate quittingby creating a smoke-free office environment that reflects positive health practices. Office personnel should remove all ashtrays and place "Thank you for not smoking" signs or other "low-key" antismoking messages in the reception area. Generally, overt scare approaches to cessation are both inappropriate and ineffective.Clinicians should document the tobacco-use status of every patient (the "ask" part of the Five A's) because all smokers and smokeless tobacco should be systematically identified and advised to quit. If requested, these individuals need to be offered brief basic cessation treatment during each office visit. More specific intervention should be targeted at tobacco users who are at high risk, for example, children or young adults who have recently started using tobacco, periodontal patients, candidates for dental implants, heavy alcohol users, periodontal patients, candidates for dental implants, heavy alcohol users, individuals who have previously been diagnosed with leukoplakia or oral cancer, pregnant women, and patients who are treatment planned to receive oral surgery. Brief cessation counseling sessions (even as short as 3 minutes) during each dental appointment can be effective. More intense treatment produces an increasing likelihood of long-term abstinence from tobacco. It is both appropriate and legal for dentists to use US Food and Drug Administration (FDA-approved nicotine replacement therapy (including nicotine patches, gum, lozenges and nicotine nasal spray) to help their patients quit using tobacco. Additionally, dental professionals should offer continued cessation support and follow-up for their patients who have decided to quit using tobacco.

Definition of Tobacco Counseling under Dental Code #01320

Under this code, tobacco cessation counseling is defined as the act of giving specific advice and practical guidance in helping an interested, generally healthy individual to quit the use of smoke and/or smokeless tobacco. Counseling strategies and formats, delivered either individually or in groups, can include the use of problem identification, problem solving, stress coping skills, weight control concepts, skills development, educational materials, self-help ideas, and relapse prevention techniques. The provision of continuing social support, care, and encouragement by the counselor(s) is essential in the effectiveness of a tobacco cessation program.

Scope of Those Who Receive Tobacco Cessation Counseling in Dental Practice under Dental Code #01320

Under this code, all smokers or smokeless tobacco users who cannot quit on their own but who desire to do so, are eligible for intensive tobacco cessation treatment and follow-up care by dental healthcare providers. More heavily addicted smokers and smokeless tobacco users and those who have underlying emotional problems (such as major depressive disorders) need to be referred to specialists who routinely assess and treat severely addicted tobacco users. In certain instances, patients who receive medication from their primary care physician can later be treated by dental personnel.

PROVISION OF COUNSELING SERVICES

In offering tobacco cessation counseling, the dental professional:

- Identifies and documents the oral conditions associated with patient's tobacco use.

- Relates this information directly to the patient, preferably by visualizing using a hand mirror, intraoral photographs, radiographs, and a periodontal probe.

- Assesses the patient's degree of addiction to tobacco products and his or her stage of readiness to quit by using biologic monitoring, that is, by means of a carbon monoxide breath analyzer, or by administering paper-and-pencil tests using appropriate forms and questionnaires.

- Provides basic information about smoking and successful quitting, stressing the reversibility of most tobacco-related disorders (participants who are motivated to quit will be asked to set a quit date within the near future, preferably two weeks).

- Cooperatively develops, with the patients, a realistic individualized treatment plan using multiple cessation strategies that deal with the social, psychological, and physiologic aspects of nicotine addiction.

Individual and/or group counseling techniques can be employed. FDA-approved nicotine replacement therapy (e.g., the use of nicotine gum, patches, nicotine nasal sprays) should be offered to virtually every smoker, except to those who have medical contraindications. To monitor progress and prevent relapse, clinicians should continue to provide social support, skills training, and follow-up. Patients should be offered ongoing problem-solving strategies related to concerns and worries about the quit process, for example, weight and stress control issues, the anticipation and avoidance of potential relapse situations in their environment (ie, being around other smokers or alcohol drinkers), and other situations unique to the person recovering from tobacco use.

FINANCIAL REIMBURSEMENT

There is no universally accepted fee schedule for tobacco cessation services that are delivered by oral health providers. Logically, tobacco counseling fees could be:

- Included in the overall charge for dental services to be rendered as listed in the treatment plan (i.e., when periodontal therapy is being considered, a clearly identified smoking cessation fee could be listed in the plan).

- Charged on a per-appointment basis (i.e., $25–100 per appointment).

- Assessed with a one-time fee for the entire anticipated counseling process ($150–500).

- Charged to medical code 305.1 "Nicotine Dependence" (from the fourth edition of the Diagnostic and Statistical Manual of Mental Disorders) using #99242 (Initial Evaluation) and #90841 (Follow-up Counseling).

Some practitioners have reported that about one-third of third-party payers (managed care) are covering smoking cessation services. Various carriers will pay for the use of nicotine replacement products by the patient but not for the counseling services.

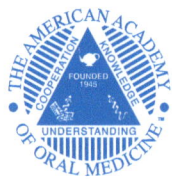

Appendix

USEFUL RESOURCES IN TOBACCO CESSATION ON THE INTERNET	
Name	*Address*
Office on Smoking and Health Reports	www.cdc.gov/tobacco
State and other data summaries	www.cdc.gov/nccdphp/osh/tobacco.htm
Tobacco and other drugs—National Institute of Drug Abuse	www.drugabuse.gov
Surgeon General's Report, 1989, Chapter 2	www.cdc.gov/tobacco/sgr/sgr_1989/1989SGRChapter2.pdf
American Lung Association	www.lungusa.org/tobacco/index/html or www.smokesignals.org
American Cancer Society	www.cancer.org
American Legacy Foundation	www.americanlegacy.org
Don't Get Sucked in—a multimedia shockwave site	www.dontgetsuckedin.com
Food and Drug Administration: Children and Tobacco	www.fda.gov/opacom/campaigns/tobacco.html
Tobacco and the Elderly	www.tcsg.org/tobacc.htm List-serv agingtob-talk@smokescreen.org
National Spit Tobacco Education Program	www.nstep.org
Oral Health America Foundation	www.oralhealthamerica.org
Program Against Teen Chewing	www.patchproject.org
Centers for Disease Control and Prevention: Health Communications Research: HealthCom Key	www.cdc.gov/od/oc/hcomm/hcomm_about.html
National Cancer Institute	www.cancer.gov
Tobacco Control Research Branch	www.dccps.nci.nih.gov/tcrb
Tobacco Control Research Branch project information	www.dccps.nci.nih.gov/tcrb/scrfa.htm
Society for Research on Nicotine and Tobacco	www.srnt.org
American Dental Association	www.ada.org (click "research" or "clinical issues" to "topical index: tobacco and nicotine")
American Dental Schools Association	ADSA-TFI@www.adsa.jhu.edu
American Medical Association—Archives of Family Medicine Clinical Review	http://archfami.ama-assn.org/issues/v9n3/full/fcr9009.html
National Oral Health Clearinghouse: spit tobacco, oral cancer	www.aerie.com/nohicweb
Spit Tobacco Prevention Network	http://home.flash.net/~stopn
Tobacco Control Resource— Indiana University	http://iumeded.med.iupui.edu
US Tobacco Cessation Programs	www.lungcheck.org
Management and Financing Cessation	www.aahp.org/atmc.htm

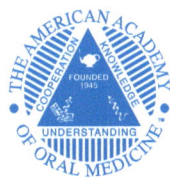

References

- American Cancer Society. 2002. "American Cancer Society guidelines for the early detection of cancer." *CA Cancer J Clin* 52(1):8-22

- American Lung Association. "Lung Cancer Fact Sheet." lung. org http://www.lung.org/lung-health-and-diseases/lung-disease-lookup/lung-cancer/learn-about-lung-cancer/lung-cancer-fact-sheet.html. (accessed November 5, 2016).

- Baker F., S. Ainsworth, J. Dye, et al. 2000. "Health risks associated with cigar smoking." *JAMA* 284:735–40.

- Barbour S.E., K. Nakashima, J.B. Zhang, et al. 1997. "Tobacco and smoking: environmental factors that modify the host response (immune system) and have an impact on periodontal health." *Crit Rev Oral Biol Med* 8:437–60.

- Barry J., K. Meade, E.G. Nabel, et al. 1989. "Effect of smoking on the activity of ischemic heart disease." *JAMA* 261:398–402.

- Bartecchi C.E., T.D. Mackenzie, and R.W. Schrier. 1994. "The human costs of tobacco use." *N Engl J Med* 330:907–12.

- Bertazzo-Silveira E., C.M. Kruger, I.P. De Toledo, A.L. Porporatti, B. Dick, C. Flores-Mir, and G. De Luca Canto. 2015. "Association between sleep bruxism and alcohol, caffeine, tobacco and drug abuse." *J Am Dent Assoc* 147 (11): 859-866

- Brandon T.H., A.T. Tiffany, K.M. Obremski, and T.N. Baker. 1990. "Post-cessation cigarette use: the process of relapse." *Addict Behav* 15:105–14.

- Burgan S. 1997. "The role of tobacco use in periodontal diseases: a literature review." *Gen Dent* 45:449–60.

- Castellsague X., N. Munoz, E. De Stefani, et al. 2000. "Smoking and drinking cessation and risk of esophageal cancer (Spain)." *Cancer Causes Control*. 11(9):813-8.

- Cahill K., S. Stevens, R. Perera, and T. Lancaster. 2013. "Pharmacological interventions for smoking cessation: an overview and network meta-analysis." *CochraneDatabase of Systematic Reviews Issue 5*. Art.No.:CD009329.DOI: 10.1002/14651858. CD009329.pub2.

- Centers for Disease Control and Prevention. 2014. "Current Cigarette Smoking Among Adults—United States, 2005-2013." *MMWR* 63:1108-1112.

- Centers for Disease Control and Prevention. 1990. "Cigarette smoking-attributable mortality and years of potential life lost in the United States." *MMWR Morb Mortal Wkly Rep 1993*; 42(33):645–9.

- Centers for Disease Control and Prevention. 2001. "State-Specific Prevalence of Current Cigarette Smoking Among Adults, and Policies and Attitudes About Secondhand Smoke—United States, 2000." *MMWR Morb Mortal Wkly Rep* 50(49):1101-6.

- Centers for Disease Control and Prevention. "Health Effects of Cigarette Smoking." cdc.gov https://www.cdc.gov/tobacco/data_statistics/fact_sheets/health_effects/effects_cig_smoking/#adults. (accessed November 5, 2016).

- Chao A., M.J. Thun, E.J. Jacobs, et al. 2000. "Cigarette smoking and colorectal cancer mortality in the cancer prevention study II." *J Natl Cancer Inst* 92:1888–96.

- Christen A.G., and E.D. Glover. 1987. "History of smokeless tobacco use in the United States." *Health Educ* 18(3):6–11.

- Christen A.G., S.J. Jay, and J.A. Christen. 2003. "Tobacco cessation and nicotine replacement therapy for dentalpractice." *General Dentistry* 51(6):525–32.

- Collins F.M. 2010. "Tobacco cessation and the impact of tobacco use on oral health." *Dental Economics February (insert)*, 100 (2): 105-115 www.ineedce.com

- Davis J.M., M.R. Arnette, J. Loewen, L. Romito and S.C. Goron. 2016. "Tobacco dependence and education: A survey of US and Canadian Dental Schools." *J Am Dent Assoc* 147 (6): 405-412

- DeHertog S.A.E., C.A.H. Wensveen, M.T. Bastiaens, et al. 2001. *J Clin Oncol* 19:231–8.

- Denisco R.C., et. al. 2011. "Prevention of prescription opioid abuse: The role of the dentist." *J Am Dent Assoc* 142 (7): 800-810

- Djordjevic M.V., D. Hoffmann, T. Glynn, and G.N. Connolly. 1995. "US commercial brands of moist snuff, 1994. I. Assessment of nicotine, moisture, and pH." *Tobacco Control* 4:62–6.

- Dowst-Myo L. 2016. "Puff, not the magic dragon: the cost of America's tobacco use. A peer-reviewed PennWell publication." *Dental Economics* March 106 (3): 92-96 www.ineedce.com

- Eberman K.M., C.A. Patten, and L.C. Dale. 1998. "Counseling patients to quit smoking, what to say, when to say it, and how to use your time to advantage." *Postgrad Med* 104:89–94.

- Encyclopedia Britannica. Chicago: 1981. p. 464–7. "Tobacco production."

- English J.P., F.A. Willius, and J. Berkston. 1940. "Tobacco and coronary disease." *JAMA* 115:1327–9.

- Environmental Protection Agency. 1992. "Respiratory health effects of passive smoking: lung cancer and other disorders." Washington (DC): Office of Health and Environmental Assessment.

- Fiore M.C., D.K. Hatsukami, and T.B. Baker. 2002. "Effective tobacco dependence treatment." *JAMA* 288:1768–71.

- Fried J.L. 2001. "The tobacco using client: clinical issues." *J Mass Dent Soc* 50(1):14–8.

- Geisler J., I.H. Omsjo, S.L. Helle, et al. 1999. "Plasma estrogen fractions in postmenopausal women receiving hormone replacement therapy: influence of route of administration and cigarette smoking." *J Endocrinol* 162:265–70.

- Grossi S.G., R.J. Genco, E.E. Machtei, et al. 1995. "Assessment of risk for periodontal disease. II. Risk indicators for alveolar bone loss." *J Periodontol* 66:23–9.

- Grossi S.G., J.J. Zambon, A.W. Ho, et al. 1994. "Assessment of risk for periodontal disease. I. Risk indicators for attachment loss." *J Periodontol* 65:260–7.

- Haber J., J. Wattles, M. Crowley, et al. 1993. "Evidence for cigarette smoking as a major risk factor for periodontitis." *J Periodontol* 64:16–23.

- Hallstrom A.P., L.A. Cobb, and R. Ray. 1986. "Smoking as a risk factor for recurrence of sudden cardiac arrest." *N Engl J Med* 314:271-5.

- Hanioka T., M. Tanaka, K. Takaya, et al. Pocket oxygen tension in smokers and non-smokers with periodontal disease. J Periodontol 2000;71:550–4.

- Harrison R., and D. Hicklin. 2015. "Electronic cigarette explosions involving the oral cavity." *J Am Dent Assoc* 147 (11): 891-896

- Hays J.T., L.C. Dale, and I.T. Croghan. 1998. "Trends in smoking related diseases, why smoking cessation is still the best medicine." *Postgrad Med* 104:56–71.

- Healthline. "COPD by the Numbers: Facts, Statistics and You." Healthline.com http://www.healthline.com/health/copd/facts-statistics-infographic#6. (accessed November 5, 2016).

- Hedin C.A., and A. Larson. 1984. "The ultrastructure of the gingival epithelium in smoker's melanosis." *J Periodontol Res* 19:177–90.

- Henningfield J.E., R.V. Fant, and S.L. Tomar. 1997. "Smokeless tobacco: an addictive drug." *Adv Dent Res* 11:330–5.

- Henningfield J.E., A. Radzins, and E.J. Cone. 1995. "Estimation of available nicotine content of six smokeless tobacco products." *Tobacco Control* 4:57–61.

- Ho K., and H.M. Abourjaily. 2001. "Pharmacological aids for smoking cessation." *J Mass Dent Soc* 50(1):30–3.

- Hoffman D., and M.V. Djordjevic. 1997. "Chemical composition and carcinogenicity of smokeless tobacco." *Adv Dent Res* 11:322–9.

- International Agency for Research on Cancer. *IARC monographs on the evaluation of carcinogenic risks to humans 54.* 2002. Lyon: IARC.

- Johnson N. 2001. "Tobacco use and oral cancer: a global perspective." *J Dent Educ* 65:328–39.

- Kabani S., G. Gallagher, and S. Frankl. 2001. "Smoking-associated oral pathoses." *J Mass Dent Soc* 50(1):8–12.

- Kazor C., G.W. Taylor, and W.J. Loesche. 1999. "The prevalence of BANA-hydrolyzing periodontopathic bacteria in smokers." *J Clin Periodontol* 26:814–21.

- Kraal J.H., and E.B. Kenney. 1979. "The response of polymorphonuclear leukocytes to chemotactic stimulation for smokers and nonsmokers." *J Periodontol Res* 14:282–9.

- Krall E.A., A.J. Garvey, and R.I. Garcia. 1999. "Alveolar bone loss in male cigar and pipe smokers." *J Am Dent Assoc* 130:57–64.

- Krupski W.C. 1987. "The peripheral vascular consequences of smoking." *Ann Vasc Surg* 5:291–304.

- Kuang J., Z. Jiang, Y. Chen, et al. 2016. "Smoking exposure and survival of patients with esophagus cancer: a systematic review and meta-analysis." *Gastroenterol Res Pract* 7682387.

- Kullo I.J., and T.W. Rooke. 2016. "Peripheral Artery Disease." *N Engl J Med* 374(9):861-71.

- Little J.W., D.A. Falace, C.S. Miller, and N.L. Rhodus. 2008. *Dental management of the medically compromised patient. 7th ed.* St. Louis: Mosby.

- Loesche W.J., W.A. Bretz, D. Kerschensteiner, et al. 1990. "Development of a diagnostic test for anaerobic periodontal infections based on plaque hydrolysis of benzoyl-DL-arginine-napththylamide." *J Clin Microbiol* 28:1551–9.

- MacFarlane G.D., M.C. Herzberg, L.F. Wolff, and N.A. Hardie. 1992. "Refractory periodontitis associated with abnormal polymorphonuclear leukocyte phagocytosis and cigarette smoking." *J Periodontol* 63:908–13.

- Mandel I. 1994. "Smoke signals: an alert for oral disease." *J Am Dent Assoc* 125:872–8.

- Mashberg A., and A.M. Samit. 1993. *Early detection, diagnosis and management of oral and oropharyngeal cancer.* New York: American Cancer Society.

- McBride P.E. 1992. "The health consequences of smoking: cardiovascular diseases." *Med Clin North Am* 76:333–53.

- Mitchell B.E., H.L. Sobel, and M.H. Alexander. 1999. "The adverse health effects of tobacco and tobacco related substances." *Primary Care* 26:463–98.

- Mohammad A. 2005. *Tobacco cessation: how to help patients quit smoking and integrate cessation into your dental practice. 2nd ed. 2.*

- Mohammad A.R. 2001. *How to help your dental patient quit smoking and integrate tobacco cessation into your dental practice: a text monograph and CD-ROM program. 1st ed.* Columbus: The Ohio State University Publication.

- Mosely L.H., F. Finseth, and M. Goody. 1978. "Nicotine and its effect on wound healing." *Plast Reconstr Surg* 61:570–5.

- Munshi T., C.J. Hickman, and S. Darlow. 2015. "Association between tobacco waterpipe smoking and head and neck conditions." *J Am Dent Assoc* 146 (10): 760-766

- Murray C.J.L., and A.D. Lopez. 1997. "Alternative projections of mortality and disability by cause 1990–2020: Global Burden of Disease Study." *Lancet* 349:1498–504.

- Muscat J.E., R.E. Harris, N.J. Haley, and E.L. Wynder. 1991. "Cigarette smoking and plasma cholesterol." *Am Heart J* 121:141–7.

- National Cancer Institute. "Cancer Stat Facts: Oral Cavity and Pharynx Cancer." seer.cancer.com http://seer.cancer.gov/statfacts/html/oralcav.html. (accessed October 30, 2016).

- National Cancer Institute. "Health effects of exposure to environmental tobacco smoke: the report of the California Environmental Protection Agency. Smoking and tobacco monograph no. 10. Bethesda, MD: US Department of Health and Human Services, National Institutes of Health, National Cancer Institute; 1999." *NIH Publication No.*: 99-4645.

- National Institute of Health, National Cancer Institute. 1997. NIH Publication No.: 97-4213. "Changes in cigarette-related disease risks and their implication for prevention and control." 2002. *CA Cancer J Clin* 52(1).

- Neugut A.I., and M.B. Terry. 2000. "Cigarette smoking and microsatellite instability: causal pathway or marker-defined subset of colon tumors." *J Natl Cancer Inst* 92:1791–3.

- Neville B.W., D.D. Damm, C.M. Allen, and C.C. Chi. 2016. *Oral and maxillofacial pathology. 4th edition.* St. Louis, Mo.: Elsevier

- Noel J.K., V.W. Rees, and G.N. Connolly. 2011. "Electronic cigarettes: a new "tobacco" industry." *Tobacco Control* 20 (1) 18. Epub 2010 Oct 7

- Pabst M.J., K.M. Pabst, J.A. Collier, et al. 1995. "Inhibition of neutrophil and monocyte defensive functions by nicotine." *J Periodontol* 66:1047–55.

- Pacifici R. 1996. "Estrogen, cytokines, and pathogenesis of postmenopausal osteoporosis." *J Bone Miner Res* 11:1043–51.

- Polosa R., B. Rodu, P. Caponnetto, M. Maglia, and C. Raciti. 2013. "A fresh look at tobacco harm reduction: the case for electronic cigarette." *Harm Reduction Journal* 10 (19): 1-11

- Quinn S.M., J.B. Zhang, J.C. Gunsolley, et al. 1996. "Influence of smoking and race on immunoglobulin G subclass concentrations in early-onset periodontitis patients." *Infect Immun* 64:2500–5.

- Regezi J.A., J.J. Sciubba, and R.C.K. Jordan. 2012. *Oral Pathology: Clinical Pathologic Correlations. 6th edition.* St. Louis, Mo.: Elsevier

- Seeman E. 1996. "The effects of tobacco and alcohol use on bone." In: Marcus R, Feldman D, Kelsey J, editors. *Osteoporosis.* Sydney: Academic Press; p. 577–97.

- Shah P.K., and R.H. Helfant. 1988. "Smoking and coronary artery disease." *Chest* 94:449–52.

- Slattery M.L., K. Curtin, K. Anderson, et al. 2000. "Association between cigarette smoking, lifestyle factors, and microsatellite instability in colon tumors." *J Natl Cancer Inst* 92:831–5.

- Smith E.A., W.S.C. Poston, C.K. Haddock, and R.E. Malone. 2016. "Installation tobacco control programs in the U.S. military." *Military Medicine* 181: 596-601

- Sugiishi M., and F. Takatsu. 1993. "Cigarette smoking is a major risk factor for coronary spasm." *Circulation* 87:76–9.

- Tipton D.A., and M.K. Dabbous. 1995. "Effects of nicotine on proliferation and extracellular matrix production of human gingival fibroblasts in vitro." *J Periodontol* 66:1056–64.

- Tomar S.L., and S. Asma. 2000. "Smoking-attributable periodontits in the United States: findings from NHANES III. National Health and Nutrition Examination Survey." *J Periodontol* 71:743–51.

- Tomar S.L., C.H. Fox, and G.N. Connolly. 2015. "Electronic cigarettes: The tobacco industry's latest threat to oral health? Guest Editorial" *J Am Dent Assoc* 146 (9): 651-653

- Uanerich D.T., W.D. Thompson, L.R. Varela, et al. 1990. "Lung cancer and exposure to tobacco smoke in the household." *N Engl J Med* 323:632–6.

- US Department of Health and Human Services. 1998. "Cigars: health effects and trends." Bethesda, MD: US Department of Health and Human Services, National Cancer Institute, Smoking and Tobacco Control Program; DHHS Publication No.: 98-4302.

- US Department of Health and Human Services. 2000. *Healthy people 2010. 2nd ed.* Washington, DC: US Department of Health and Human Services.

- US Department of Health and Human Services. 1989. "Reducing the health consequences of smoking: 25 years of progress: a report of the surgeon general." Rockville, MD. DHHS Publication No.: 98-8411.

- US Department of Health and Human Services. 1986. "The health consequences of using smokeless tobacco. A report of the advisory committee to the surgeon general." Bethesda, MD: Public Health Service, National Institutes of Health; NIH Publication No.: 86-2874.

- US Department of Health and Human Services. 2014. Printed with corrections, January 2014. "The Health Consequences of Smoking – 50 Years of Progress. A Report of the Surgeon General." Atlanta, GA: US Dept of Health and Human Services, Centers for Disease Control and Prevention, National Center for Chronic Disease Prevention and Health Promotion, Office on Smoking and Health.

- Warnakulasuriya S., W..J. Newell, and I. van der Waal. 2007. "Nomenclature and classification of potentially malignant disorders of the oral mucosa." *J Oral Pathol Med* 36: 575-80.

- Winn D.M. 1997. "Epidemiology of cancer and other systemic effects associated with the use of smokeless tobacco." *Adv Dent Res* 11:313–21.

- Women and smoking: a report of the surgeon general. 2002. *MMWR Morb Mortal Wkly Rep* 51(RR-12).

- World Health Organization (WHO): Tobacco Fact Sheet N339 2011

- Wray A., and W.F. McGuirt. 1993. "Smokeless tobacco usage associated with oral carcinoma." *Arch Otolaryngol Head Neck Surg* 119(9):929–93.

- Wyss A.B., M. Hashibe, Y.A. Lee, et al. 2016 Oct 15. "Smokeless Tobacco Use and the Risk of Head and Neck Cancer: Pooled Analysis of US Studies in the INHANCE Consortium." *Am J Epidemiol.*

- Zambon J.J., S.G. Grossi, E.E. Machtei, et al. 1996. "Cigarette smoking increases the risk for subgingiva infection with periodontal pathogens." *J Periodontol* 67:1050–4.

- Zhang Y. 2013. "Epidemiology of esophageal cancer." *World J Gastroenterol* 19(34):5598-5606.

TEXTBOOKS

- *ADA Practical Guide to Patients with Medical Conditions*. 2012. American Dental Association. Wiley Blackwell

- *ADA/PDR Guide To Dental Therapeutics (Fifth Edition)*. 2009. ADA Publishing Division. Thompson PDR

- Little J.W., D.A. Falace, C.S. Miller, and N.L. Rhodus. 2008. *Dental Management of the Medically Compromised Patient (Seventh Edition)*. St Louis: Mosby.

- O'Neil, M., ed. 2015. *The ADA Practical Guide to Substance Abuse Disorders and Safe Prescribing* (Chapter 7) .American Dental Association. WILEY Blackwell

- Wynn R.L., T.F. Meiller, and H.L. Crossley. 2010-2011. *Drug Information Handbook for Dentistry (Sixteenth Edition)*. Lexi-Comp, Inc.

ADA PDF SOURCES

- ADA Guide Smoking Cessation
- ADA Guide Smok-less Cessation

PATIENT INFORMATION

- American Lung Association: www.lung.org
- America Heart Association: www.heart.org
- BecomeAnEx: www.bceomeanex.org
- Quitnet by me you health: www.quitnet.com
- Centers for Disease Control and Prevention "Tips From Former Smokers" campaign to educate the public on the dangers of tobacco. Toll-free quit line number, 1-800-QUIT-NOW.
- There is also help available at 1-800-QUITNOW (1-800-784-8669) or www.smokefree.gov5, where counselors can advise smokers on the best treatment options for them.

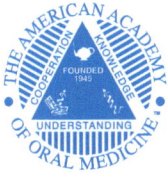

The American Academy of Oral Medicine
2150 N. 107th St., Suite 205
Seattle, Washington 98133
PHONE: (206) 209-5279 · EMAIL: info@aaom.com

Application for AAOM Membership

ELIGIBILITY FOR MEMBERSHIP

1. Nominee for **Regular Membership** shall be a graduate of an accredited Dental School or Medicine School and shall be a member of his/her representative National Society and shall pursue special interest or accomplishment in the field of Oral Medicine.

2. Nominee for **Affiliate Membership** (student) shall be a graduate of an accredited Dental or Medical School and shall be a member of his/her representative National Society and currently in training in a Postdoctoral program.

3. Nominee for **Student Membership** shall be a student currently enrolled in a pre-doctoral program in an accredited dental or medical school. Students are those seeking a DDS, DMD or MD degree.

4. The fiscal year for dues starts January 1.

5. After acceptance into the Academy, Active Membership dues are paid annually and include a subscription to ORAL SURGERY, ORAL MEDICINE, ORAL PATHOLOGY, ORAL RADIOLOGY, and ENDODONTOLOGY.

6. Please see the AAOM website for more membership information and how to apply: www.aaom.com.

www.ingramcontent.com/pod-product-compliance
Lightning Source LLC
Chambersburg PA
CBHW041452210326
41599CB00004B/220